Beginnings Count

The Twentieth Century Fund sponsors and supervises timely analyses of economic policy, foreign affairs, and domestic political issues. Not-for-profit and nonpartisan, the Fund was founded in 1919 and endowed by Edward A. Filene.

Beginnings Count

THE TECHNOLOGICAL
IMPERATIVE IN AMERICAN
HEALTH CARE

David J. Rothman

A Twentieth Century Fund Book

New York   Oxford
OXFORD UNIVERSITY PRESS
1997

Oxford University Press

Oxford   New York
Athens   Auckland   Bangkok   Bogota   Bombay   Buenos Aires
Calcutta   Cape Town   Dar es Salaam   Delhi   Florence   Hong Kong
Istanbul   Karachi   Kuala Lumpur   Madras   Madrid   Melbourne
Mexico City   Nairobi   Paris   Singapore   Taipei   Tokyo   Toronto

and associated companies in
Berlin   Ibadan

Copyright © 1997 by Oxford University Press

Published by Oxford University Press, Inc.
198 Madison Avenue, New York, New York 10016

Oxford is a registered trademark of Oxford University Press

All rights reserved. No part of this publication may be reproduced,
stored in a retrieval system, or transmitted, in any form or by any means,
electronic, mechanical, photocopying, recording or otherwise,
without the prior permission of Oxford University Press.

Library of Congress Cataloging-in-Publication Data
Rothman, David J.
Beginnings count :
The technological imperative in American health care /
David J. Rothman.
p.   cm.   "A Twentieth Century Fund book."
Includes bibliographical references and index.
Other title: American values, medical technologies, and health care policy.
ISBN 0-19-511118-4
1. Medical policy—United States.   2. Medical technology—United States.
3. Insurance, Health—United States.   4. Health services accessibility—United States.
5. Medical care—United States—Public opinion.
6. Middle class—United States—Attitudes.
I. Title.   [DNLM: 1. Delivery of Health Care—history—United States.
2. Health Policy—history—United States.   3. Insurance, Health—United States.
4. Social Values—United States.   5. Technology, Medical—United States.
W 84 AA1 R8b 1997]   RA395.A3R68   1997
362.1'0973—dc21   DNLM/DLC   for Library of Congress   96-46368

987654321

Printed in the United States of America
on acid-free paper

TO ARYEH NEIER
For Leading the Way

Foreword

Despite all our protests to the contrary, inequality is a widespread American phenomenon. We declare formal allegiance to the concept of equality, but we accept a greater degree of difference in the conditions that prevail in almost every area of life than does any other advanced nation. For example, we endorse, and indeed lately have been reenforcing, an economic system that produces unusually unequal results in terms of income and wealth; indeed, we celebrate the accumulation of vast fortunes by individuals. We carry this even further by our reluctance to provide public sector support to meet the needs that result from this inequality.

We have found it remarkably easy to accustom ourselves to the presence of homeless people on the streets of our cities, while refusing to support low-income housing and extending new tax breaks to those who sell expensive homes. We shed the burden of welfare, and waffle about education and training programs. In all too many areas in fact, we choose public services that are substandard for a modern nation because they cost less. When it comes to health care, our attitudes are even more difficult to comprehend.

We brag about our health care system—the most modern, technologically advanced system in the world. We want the best, risk-free care available when we need it. At the same time, we wear blinders when it comes to the truth that the kind of health care we want is so extraordinarily expensive that, as currently structured, it means that the treatment available to people at different levels of society is far from equal. Approximately 40 million of our citizens are not covered for the costs of care—a situation that is not countenanced in any other advanced nation. In the case of health care, as in so many other areas, the truth is we want what we want, but we do not want to pay to ensure that others also have what they need.

What makes the issue more complex is that the politics of health care are so obscure that it is dangerous for anyone to talk about the real trade-offs between costs and benefits. We claim that we are willing to live with the outcomes the market produces, but clearly the way we have structured the health care program that most affects the middle class—Medicare—suggests that this is not the case. The debates that are developing as our nation faces the increasingly difficult job of meeting the health needs of an aging population will be an interesting test of our willingness to live with the result of market forces. It is one thing to leave the bottom 20 percent out of the system; it would be quite another, politically, to say that only the top 20 percent can afford the best health care that is available—and so be it.

Although the dilemma we face is seldom explicitly discussed, it is at the heart of the current health care crisis in the United States. The great virtue of David J. Rothman's book is that he confronts the contradictions, using as his starting point high-cost medical technologies. This approach allows him to bring into play most of the factors that influence the shape of the health care delivery systems in the United States. Moreover, most of the current issues, public and private, flow from our desire to use these technologies to their fullest.

Rothman's analysis starts with an exploration of the three great historical struggles over health care that marked this century: the effort during the New Deal, which culminated in the development of non-governmental but still non-profit health insurance, Blue Cross and Blue Shield; the one great federal assumption of health care responsibility—the enactment of Medicare for the elderly in 1965; and the Clinton health care program that went down in a flurry of negative advertising. Each of these struggles is illuminated by a close look at the history of an important technology that represented a microcosm of the issues involved in the larger forces at work during that period. Thus the development of the iron lung, the dialysis machine, and the respirator have raised all too often unarticulated and yet fundamental questions that underlie the larger public debates about health care.

Rothman shows that the middle-class desire for the most sophisticated health care available no matter what the cost, combined with the political power of that group, is the defining influence on what actually takes place. The story tells us a lot about how we got where we are today and perhaps even more about the current impasse concerning how to pay for health care.

The Twentieth Century Fund has a long history of looking at both health care and the social responsibilities of our society. In the area of health care, we have supported, among others, *Unloving Care*, Bruce Vladeck's landmark examination of nursing homes; *Profit Motive and Patient Care*, Bradford Gray's study of hospital accountability and responsibility; *The Most Useful Gift*, Jeffrey Prottas' examination of organ transplant policy; and *Beyond Medicare*, Malvin Schechter's look at the costs of providing care to the oldest of our citizens. We have also supported explorations of the difficult issues involved in the very basic issue of equality of access to basic services in studies such as Ken Rosen's *Affordable Housing*; Peter Rossi's *Without Shelter*; a Task Force on affordable housing; Andrew Achenbaum's *Social Security*; and our Basics series, which has looked at Social Security, Medicare, Welfare, and Medicaid. Indeed, we consider these issues so important that we have numerous studies in these areas under way, such as James Galbraith's exploration of the inequality crisis in America and Theda Skocpol's study of the problems of meeting the demands of old and young.

Rothman has provided us with an opportunity to explore yet another facet of this complicated issue of need and cost and the American willingness to shoulder the burden of making them match. We are grateful to him.

Richard C. Leone, President
The Twentieth Century Fund
January 1997

Acknowledgments

In the course of thinking about and writing this book, I incurred several debts that I am pleased to acknowledge. The Twentieth Century Fund encouraged me to bring history to bear on questions of health policy, and its generous support facilitated the effort. For much of the period, a good friend (and former student), Ellen Chesler, was at the Fund and her many insightful comments and critiques were always helpful. I adopted practically every one of her suggestions and the book is much better for it. I profited, as well, from the comments of Jeffrey House, my editor at Oxford, and his oversight of the manuscript.

I had the occasion to present in preliminary form some of the materials in the book and the exchanges that followed were invariably useful. I was first attracted to the Blue Cross story because of an imaginative project organized by Daniel Fox; a number of historians and political scientists each explored a facet of the history of New York's Blue Cross and then came together to discuss their methodologies and findings. It was interdisciplinary work at its best and a model worth emulating. I also presented an overview of my work at a conference on health care policy organized by James Morone, and again, the contributions of other scholars and their comments on my approach were very useful. Over the period, I enjoyed the many substantive and editorial comments that came from Robert Silvers, editor of the New York Review of Books where part of Chapter Five originally appeared.

I must thank, too, the librarians and archivists at Empire Blue Cross, the March of Dimes, the New York Academy of Medicine, and the Columbia College of Physicians and Surgeons for their unfailing courtesies. I had the advantage of the research skills of a group of Columbia undergraduates and graduate students, each more energetic and diligent than the other.

They include Aina Lakus, Rebekah Gee, Jennifer Geetter, Zachary Meisel, and Martin Rivlin. Colleagues at the Center for the Study of Society and Medicine were always ready to listen to initial formulations and suggest useful research strategies to pursue.

I benefited greatly from an extraordinarily comprehensive review of the manuscript by Deborah Stone. She not only highlighted weaknesses in the argument, but went on to suggest ways of strengthening points that she intuited or knew I wanted to make.

Finally, I have the pleasure, once again, of acknowledging the contributions of Sheila Rothman. She moves comfortably between past and present, and encourages me to do likewise. She sets a tone, both at home and in the Center, that gives high priority to research and writing. It has influenced the careers of Matthew and Micol, and continues to shape mine as well.

Barnard, Vermont   D. J. R.
December 1996

Contents

Beginnings Count

Introduction

The starting point for this book rests in my ongoing puzzlement and fascination with the question of why the American health care system is so highly idiosyncratic. Although the notion of American exceptionalism can be exaggerated, among Western countries American medicine stands out as practically unique. No matter what the yardstick, the differences are profound. Compared to other industrialized countries, the United States trains a greater percentage of medical specialists and subspecialists. We insist more vigorously than others on the right to choose our own doctors; we pay higher fees for each visit and procedure, in the process making American physicians the richest in the world. We invest more heavily than others in biomedical research. No other country follows medical developments as closely as we do; more medical journalists are employed in the United States than anywhere else. And as everyone knows, we devote more of our national resources to health care. It now represents a trillion-dollar industry.[1]

As remarkable as this roster is, there are two other characteristics that are even more distinctive of American health care. First, the United States will enter the twenty-first century as the only industrialized country, South Africa aside, that does not have a national health insurance system. As vital as medicine is to us, 40 million Americans have no assured access to health care. What Germany accomplished in the 1890s, England in the 1920s, and Canada in the 1960s, has still not come to pass here.

Second, American medicine is singular in its dependence on powerful and costly medical technologies. Nowhere else do physicians rely so heavily on diagnostic imaging machines (including MR and CT scanners); or have such frequent recourse to life-saving devices like dialysis machines (to treat kidney failure) and extracorporeal membrane oxygenators (to sustain newborns with underdeveloped lung capacity). Medicine in this country has already entered the twenty-first century, and to judge by the prospects in pharmacology and genetics, the wizardry is certain to continue.

The chapters that follow explore the exceptional character of American health care by examining these two phenomena in depth and exploring the crucial links between them. The impact of medical technology on all aspects of American health care cannot be exaggerated. Technology bears the heaviest responsibility for the costliness of American medicine and the magnitude of subspecialization. But the feature of technology that is most fundamental to the argument here is the degree to which the public, most notably the middle-class public, is fascinated and attracted to it, and determined to enjoy unlimited access. Americans have an extraordinary romance with medical technology, particularly when it has the capacity to save the almost moribund patient, when it comes closest to fulfilling the vision of Zachariah and giving new life to dry bones. The histories of the iron lung, in the first instance, and the kidney dialysis machine, in the second, illustrate the allure of what we might call the resurrectionist capacity of technology. These interventions are, by all meanings of the term, heroic, a label that has lately taken on something of a negative characteristic (as in, no heroic treatment please) but that originally conveyed the awesome power of the technology and the wondrous benefits which flowed from it.

This passion for technology carries implications not only for the high cost of medical care but also for limitations on its availability. As we shall see, the unwillingness to broaden access to health care is intimately related to this unconditional commitment to technology. Middle-class Americans' devotion to the machines, especially when they have life-saving capacity, underlies an ongoing refusal to socialize medical care and make it available to everyone. Because the middle classes will not tolerate restrictions on access to these technologies, the lower classes are left to fend for themselves. The truth of this statement is nowhere better evidenced than by Americans' recent unwillingness to enact national health insurance.

There is nothing new about this dynamic. Since the 1930s, health care policy in the United States has reflected the needs and concerns of the middle classes. The design evolved and justified itself in terms of giving them all the medicine they wanted, making certain that they would be able to afford the technologies that so captured their imagination. At the same time, health care policy tried to realize this commitment in ways that were most compatible with middle-class political sensibilities. Wherever possible, the system relied upon the private, not the public sector; the preference was for health insurance purchased through the marketplace, not provided by the government. At least until the passage of Medicare, in 1965, the linkage held, and the middle classes could satisfy their own desires without confronting a challenge to their political axioms. Employees of large corporations, members of well-organized unions, and those who ran small businesses could afford the premiums; generally speaking, they were not particularly concerned with health care costs. They could have it all, and not invoke the specter or the reality of big government.

These arrangements, however, came with a price—paid not by the middle classes but by the lower classes. Those who held poor-paying jobs, whether self-employed or employed by others, or who were periodically or permanently unemployed, were left to fend for themselves. To be sure, they had access to public clinics and the emergency rooms of large public hospitals, or if they were lucky, to ward beds in private voluntary hospitals; they might be able to scrape by in the event of short-term and not very serious illnesses. But let the disease be recurring or critical, and they would suffer the acute consequences of being outside a national health insurance program.

Before elaborating on this argument, a brief statement on terminology is appropriate. Although the term *middle class* may seem amorphous, it is used here to delineate social and economic characteristics, on the one hand, and a commitment to certain values, on the other. The middle classes are those who generally hold full-time employment, who run a profitable if small business, who have a skilled job in a major corporation, or who are members of a protective and powerful labor union. The values that they typically espouse include personal autonomy, personal responsibility, and personal choice; the superiority of private initiatives and voluntary associations; freedom from government regulation; and up to a point where self-interest would dictate otherwise, an absence of dependence upon government support, particularly in the realm of welfare. Clearly, there is something artificial about the term *middle class*; it is a construct of convenience, analogous to the *we* that authors make the subject of a large generalization. But it also has a social reality that must be appreciated. This reality, to cite a series of recent political advertisements sponsored by the health insurance industry, is embodied in "Harry and Louise." This fictive couple, sitting in the spacious living room of their private home, criticized many of the aspects of the Clinton heath care plan, and complacently concluded that they were much better off sticking with the insurance plan they already had. In other words, they represented the employed, insured middle class, not without their worries, but not dependent upon government largess to meet their health care needs.

Implicit in the approach taken here to health care policy—made explicit in the chapters that follow—is, first, an emphasis on the determinative role of social values, and, second, a consideration of how these values originated, evolved, and were confirmed or disconfirmed by experience. Most current discussions and analyses neglect these two elements. Take, for example, the numerous obituaries that followed the death of the Clinton national health care plan. The interplay of politics, personalities, maneuvers, and interest groups, not underlying social values, has dominated scholarly and journalistic interpretations. Bad timing, the emergence of other issues, including NAFTA and Somalia, that required the president's attention, the negative consequences of appointing the first lady to lead the campaign, the endemic difficulty of breaking through congressional gridlock, especially for a president elected by a minority of the voters, and the power of business and insurance lobbyists have all been advanced to explain why the administration's initiative was defeated.

But to focus only on individual lapses and malfeasance obscures the larger lessons to be drawn from the abortive campaign. Events in Washington make up only one part of the story. No less vital to an understanding of the design and fate of health care policies are more comprehensive considerations of how the public, essentially the middle classes, now and in the past, has conceptualized the enterprise and why it finally prefers, some notable exceptions aside, to keep government's role to a minimum. If Americans do not have national health insurance, it is because the middle classes have been unwilling to support it.

Tracing the origins and impact of social values is all the more important because in this arena, where political scientists leave off, economists take over. Their influence is not difficult to explain. The high cost of the American system brings them to the fore, in the hope that their analyses will differentiate among such critical and contributing causes as waste, greed, and inefficiency on the part of hospitals, physicians, and drug companies. Perhaps the most conspicuous economic fact about American health care is the percentage of the Gross National Product that it consumes. Even readers who follow the debate only casually know that the percentage was once 6, then 10, and now has reached 14. Some economists, only half-jokingly, plot graphs demonstrating that if current trends continue, by the year 2040 health care will take up nearly 100% of the GNP. The exercise is like charting a fever in a very sick patient—although it is too easily forgotten that on this thermometer, no one knows what normal is.

Economics has also framed a second noteworthy fact about the existing health system—that some 40 million Americans lack health insurance. By dint of bad timing, Americans have been forced to consider how to expand access to care just when they felt the need to devise strategies to reduce expenditures. Because the United States waited so long before taking up national health insurance, the issue surfaced just as medical costs were skyrocketing. Obviously, but no less portentously, the two goals are, at best, in conflict and, at worst, fundamentally incompatible.

This was not the situation that other industrialized countries confronted. Governments in Germany, England, and Canada certainly had to estimate costs and, after implementation, find ways to control expenditures. But for them, other, noneconomic values could assume greater prominence on the national agenda, including judgments about what services a government owed its citizens and what citizens owed each other.

In the United States, however, the simultaneous appearance of the questions of widening access and containing costs elevated fiscal considerations above others. It therefore requires an act of imagination to remember that GNP percentages are not the only possible index for judging the worth of a policy. One alternative, for example, might be to rely on health care outcomes, not ignoring costs but making them a second order of priority. A national debate might center on why the infant mortality rate in the United States is so high and what might be done to lower it. Or we might address the question of why the death rate in black communities like Harlem exceeds that of Bangladesh. Picture a graph that plotted rates of mortality rather than percentages of GNP and raised the question of how these rates might be decreased.

Because of the near obsession with GNP percentages, American values have been made to appear irrelevant to the process of reform. To be sure, one or another academic or politician will declare that health policy is ultimately a moral issue. But the phrase is usually invoked without meaningful elaboration, a rhetorical device more than the starting point for analysis. Indeed, public policy analysts have treated decision making in health care as if it were quite separable and distinct from social traditions. Perhaps it is because health care is already messy enough without adding to it the still more complicating elements of history; or perhaps health care, like other policy fields, breeds its own kind of insularity. But to pass over inherited ideals and preferences is to miss one of the most vital, if not always visible, determinants of policy. Perhaps this is what John Maynard Keynes had in mind when he remarked during the Great Depression: "Practical men who believe themselves to be quite exempt from any intellectual influence are usually the slaves of some defunct economist. . . . It is ideas, not vested interests, which are dangerous for good or evil."[2]

Thus, this book intends not to serve philosophical purposes, that is, conceptualizing and defining the values that should govern the politics and economics of health care, but historical purposes, to illuminate the development and import of American values in health care and the part they have played and will continue to play in the design of health care policy.

The chapters in this book explore decisive moments in the evolution of American public policy and public attitudes. They are intensive analyses of major turning points, not case studies as such. The chapters alternate in focus, looking at critical innovations in both the provision of health insurance and the use of medical technologies. This is a tale of three policies and three machines—Blue Cross, Medicare, and the (failed) Health Security Act, on the one hand, and the iron lung, the dialysis machine, and the respirator, on the other. Taken together, they enable us to grasp the complex interrelationship between social values and health policy. They help us to understand why middle-class Americans preferred to keep government out of health care, when they made exceptions to the rule, and how their preferences fit with their own experiences and served their self interest. It is lived history, not an abstract commitment to voluntary associations or the marketplace, or a reflexive opposition to big government, that has mattered most.

The story begins in the 1930s with the origins of private health insurance in the form of Blue Cross. This decade witnessed the introduction of many novel and innovative New Deal social welfare programs, including Social Security, but health care was not among them. Despite the efforts of a number of urban-based and liberal-minded Democratic congressmen, national health insurance was not enacted. Instead, a very different orientation took hold. As odd as it may seem, the lesson that Americans were taught, and learned, over the course of the Great Depression was that private hospital insurance, not government insurance, represented the American Way in health care.

The most active and effective transmitter of this message was Blue Cross. Created in the 1930s in response to the fiscal crisis that was affecting hospitals (charitable donations as well as patient admissions had dropped precipitously), Blue Cross self-consciously and successfully presented itself as the alternative to government involvement in health care. Its national and state organizations promised to give members all the hospital care they might need, in the process obviating, and impugning, the need for government intervention. Blue Cross adeptly aimed this message at the middle classes, to the distinct purpose of removing them from a potential coalition that might propel national health insurance forward. A carefully conceived and skillfully implemented strategy separated out the middle classes and won their allegiance to the principle that health insurance belonged to the private sector, not the least of the reasons being that it worked very well for them. It was a stunning accomplishment and its consequences persist to this day.

The social impact of the first life-saving medical machine, the iron lung, also framed American attitudes and policies toward the provision of health care. Developed by Philip Drinker, in 1928, the artificial breathing machine was able to sustain polio patients whose diaphragm muscles had been paralyzed by the virus. Although the technology had its scarier side (to some it was an iron cage or steel casket), its efficacy inspired an extraordinary charitable campaign to make certain that no one died for lack of access to the machine.

Over the 1930s and 1940s, the National Foundation for Infantile Paralysis (NFIP, better known as the March of Dimes) successfully disseminated this message. Like Blue Cross, it constructed and popularized a particular story, one that had critical significance for health policy. Through its fundraising appeals and the activities of its hundreds of chapter networks, it taught Americans that rationing was unacceptable, that it was unnecessary, and that private philanthropy could meet the challenge of providing services. The foundation's message was well received, helped by the fact that polio was President Franklin Delano Roosevelt's disease, and a children's disease, indeed a middle-class children's disease. With these assists, the foundation was able to fulfill its mission and inculcate an unambiguous ethos: that Americans had to democratize access to medical machines, and that the private sector was fully capable of realizing the goal.

The third critical moment in the formulation and expression of American values in health care was the 1965 enactment of Medicare—the first and to date only occasion in which the federal government underwrote the cost of health care for a significant segment of the population. From the mid-1930s until the mid-1960s, health insurance had remained, just as Blue Cross hoped and the NFIP exemplified, a private, not public, function; various congressional initiatives to expand the role of government were soundly defeated. The passage of Medicare seemed to break with tradition, but in ever so many ways it did not. Its supporters insisted that Medicare was the exception to the rule that the private sector was responsible for health insurance. Yes, the elderly required government assistance—but all others could be left to depend on the marketplace. By failing to define health care as a right due all citizens and by drawing spurious distinctions between the needs of the elderly and the ability of the young to fend for themselves, Medicare's proponents set back, indefinitely as it turns out, the movement for national health insurance.

Only by focusing on the uncompromising insistence of the middle classes to have full access to life-saving medical machines does the next critical change in health policy make sense, the 1973 provision for federal underwriting of all the costs of care for patients with end-stage kidney disease. In 1960, Belding Scribner of the University of Washington medical school devised a technique for hooking up patients suffering from kidney failure to a machine that would essentially perform the function of the kidney, cleansing the blood of its impurities. The dilemma was that the number of patients whose lives would be saved by kidney dialysis far outnumbered the available machines. To cope with the shortfall, the Seattle medical society, and similar groups in other states as well, created "Who Shall Live?" committees to select which patients would go on the machines.

The exercise of rationing by these committees spurred public indignation, which organizations like the National Association of Patients on Hemodialysis (NAPH) translated into effective lobbying. As with the iron lung, the message was that no one should be denied the benefits of a life-saving medical machine, particularly when the beneficiaries were members of the middle class—which initially was the defining social characteristic of patients undergoing dialysis. NAPH rhetoric and strategies, which included one of its members undergoing dialysis in a congressional committee room, brought this lesson home to Americans in general and the Congress in particular. Because the middle classes could not afford to purchase dialysis machines, the government was obliged to underwrite the costs. Once the line was sharply drawn between money and life, the answer in a democratically elected political forum had to be life. No politician would wish to defend the proposition that the rich could live because they had access to a machine, while the middle class died because they could not afford it. And so the 1973 amendment to Medicare provided full coverage for patients with end-stage kidney disease.

Before long, however, the underwriting of dialysis incited criticism and complaints. By 1990, the program was expending $3 billion to keep less than half a million patients alive, and a number of commentators were beginning to argue that something was dreadfully wrong with the American approach to health care, both in terms of gross expense and its unqualified commitments to machines. This revisionist outlook remained peripheral to policy until it was bolstered by the subsequent experience with the artificial ventilator. Over the 1970s and 1980s, the respirator, far more powerfully than the iron lung or the dialysis machine, provoked skeptical and hostile responses from patients as well as from physicians. A profound malaise with the machine was widespread, and one need only invoke its defining moment to confirm the point—the image of Karen Ann Quinlan, curled in fetal position and tethered to the respirator. Here was a technology that was not saving the young or the able-bodied but keeping the dead alive, and at enormous expense. Because of the respirator, we all had to suffer a $100,000 funeral.

The dissatisfaction with the respirator provoked a series of responses that aimed to set limits on the provision of medical care. Many patients scurried to write living wills and advance directives so as to avoid weeks or months on the machine. Legislatures rushed to make these documents lawful and binding on hospitals and doctors. And all the while, a new cadre of medical commentators, bioethicists, inveighed against a seemingly unquenchable thirst for medical technologies, which they often attributed to a national unwillingness to accept death. Indeed, this hostility to medical technologies seemed so persuasive and legitimate that political leaders came to believe that some type of restraint on medical services, a system of rationing (although the word itself could not be used), might be acceptable to the public. This would be the more likely if some beneficial trade-off was involved, like giving the middle class the comfort and security of national health insurance.

The Clinton administration adopted this formulation, at least part way. It proposed a program that would give the middle classes the security and savings that they seemed to want, and the lower classes the access that they needed, along with a ceiling on expenditures to control medical care costs. All the evidence suggested that the middle classes were beginning to find private insurance too expensive and arbitrary. To change jobs, to be laid off, or for that matter, to have a bout of severe illness, often resulted in a loss of coverage. Thus Clinton could serve the interests of both the middle class and the lower class.

The plan itself took shape around the concept of "managed competition," a frankly hybrid creation in which private health care plans competed for subscribers under the watchful eye of public regional alliances; marketplace mechanisms would reduce costs while government regulation would maintain quality and fairness. But to make absolutely certain that expenses did not escalate wildly, the plan included a "budget cap." Just how it would operate and whether it constituted a mechanism for rationing were questions that the Clinton administration preferred not to address. Confident that eliminating waste and bringing efficiency to health care would take care of most of the problem, the administration tried its best to bury the issue.

It was a fateful miscalculation. In effect, the Clinton team gave the rationing question over to the opposition. A diverse coalition, ranging from the religious right to fiscal conservatives, exploited the issue to the fullest; rationing became the fact that an untrustworthy administration was desperately seeking to hide. By the time critics were through, the middle classes were convinced that the new plan would bring not only higher taxes but, at least for them, significantly reduced access to medical treatment and technology. Within a few months of the plan's introduction, they deserted the administration, deciding that they were better off with what they already had, whatever the consequences for others.

For a historian to introduce a study of health policy by asserting the relevance of past events seems too predictable and self-serving. So better to allow a political scientist, Robert Putnam, to endorse this disciplinary approach. "History matters," Putnam tells us in his study of civic traditions, because social developments are "path dependent." "What comes first (even if it was in some sense 'accidental') conditions what comes later. Individuals may 'choose' their institutions, but they do not choose them under circumstances of their own making, and their choices in turn influence the rules within which their successors choose."[3] To illuminate the many meanings and implications of this process is the essential goal of this book. Put most succinctly, the pages that follow aim to demonstrate that beginnings do count.

1 Blue Cross and the American Way in Health Care

In health care as in so many other spheres, the boundary lines between private enterprise and government programs have been continually negotiated and altered. In a country that remains more complacently pragmatic than rigidly ideological, the division between what belongs to the marketplace and is assumed to be individual citizens' own responsibility (like purchasing an automobile) and what is the state's obligation to its citizens (like providing fire and police protection or, after 1935, Social Security benefits) is not so much anchored and fixed as contested and fluctuating. The outcomes reflect the values that citizens hold (for example, the elderly should not be left to fend for themselves) as well as the financial and ideological preferences of organizations, both corporate and voluntary. But there is an artificiality about such a distinction—because popularly held values affect organizational decisions, and organizations energetically attempt to shape social values.

In the ongoing demarcation of private obligations and public duties, the provision of health insurance to citizens has generally been defined as a function of the private sector. In a pattern established in the 1930s and maintained thereafter, citizens (except for the elderly and the very poor) must purchase health insurance in the marketplace, either directly or through their employer, rather than receive it as part of a package of government benefits. It is up to each one of us to protect ourselves against the financial consequences of illness.

The obvious and critical question is how did this significant division of responsibility come about? Why did insurance companies, not government financed programs, emerge to dominate the field? Why have most Americans accepted this arrangement as proper and just? To make these questions even more intriguing, this arrangement took hold in the United States in the 1930s, at the very moment when the scope of government activity was expanding most dramatically. It was at a time of maximum flexibility, when the role of government was being redefined in fundamental fashion, that the American Way in health care became private, not public. Thus, the best starting point for understanding the peculiar features of the American health care system is the Great Depression. Historically speaking, this was the decisive moment in the allocation of responsibility between the sectors.

With good reason, one might well have anticipated that the New Deal, which secured the implementation of such programs as Social Security, would also have implemented government underwriting of health care. After all, the Depression undermined the financial stability of the middle classes; the threat of downward mobility was undoubtedly more ominous in this decade than in any other. In fact, the middle classes were in so tenuous a position that governmental welfare policies underwent a striking alteration. Well into the 1930s, poor relief continued to rely upon indoor, almshouse support for the needy. These Dickensian facilities were still thriving so that the elderly and disabled poor, particularly when they were considered to be "unworthy," were housed and fed in these dingy and miserable institutions.

Over the course of the Depression, however, the almshouse fell into disrepute, replaced by such New Deal relief programs as the Works Project Administration (employing the needy on public works) and social security pensions. In fact, WPA regulations explicitly prohibited the expenditure of its funds to build or enlarge almshouses. Why the injunction? Why the abandonment, at long last, of the almshouse? Because for the first time, almshouse relief would have had to include the middle classes. With state and city budgets staggering under the burden of relief and private charities altogether unequal to the task, absent a WPA or Social Security Act, many of the now unemployed would have had to enter the almshouse. The prospect of having respectable middle-class citizens reside in such facilities was so disturbing that government relief policy was transformed.

Imagine this same dynamic at work in health care. Picture the middle classes having no alternative but to crowd into public hospitals, to receive medical services in wards crammed with 12 or 20 beds. It is not fanciful to suggest that had this been the case, intense pressure would have been exerted on the government to enact health insurance coverage, thereby enabling the middle classes to continue to use the voluntary hospital system. But the private sector self-consciously and successfully short-circuited the process. Despite the introduction of a variety of bills into Congress and some hesitant first steps, public policy did not attend to health care.

To understand this result requires an analysis not only of Washington politics (which has been carried out so well by such scholars as James Morone, Theodore Marmor, and Paul Starr) but also of developments outside the halls of Congress. In particular, it is critical to look at the development of the programs and procedures that emerged to meet the needs of the middle classes in a way that satisfied not only their pocketbooks but their consciences. It was the genius of Blue Cross to realize both agendas. In the 1930s, in state after state, its chapters implemented and promoted a plan that fulfilled the immediate requirements of the middle classes. Moreover, Blue Cross framed its approach in political terms. Its self-declared goal was not only to meet the day-to-day concerns of the middle classes, but in so doing, to remove health insurance from the national political agenda.

Before the 1930s and the rise of Blue Cross, very few Americans had prepaid insurance that covered hospital costs or doctors' bills. A number of fraternal and mutual benevolent societies, their members bound together by ties of common neighborhood, employment, or ethnicity, did provide assistance in times of illness, but it was usually cash payments to supplement family incomes when the chief breadwinner was too sick to work. In the 1910s and 1920s, when the advantages of medical care became more pronounced, some of these societies helped members to pay their medical bills, but again they did so through a cash benefit, not by arranging insurance policies. In all, the programs were limited in scope and affected very few people. Even in New York City where fraternal organizations flourished, a 1914 survey revealed that only some 170,000 persons had any type of insurance. In effect, before the Great Depression and before Blue Cross, families were on their own when it came to hospital or medical bills.[1]

Blue Cross changed all that, realizing its goals through two distinctive strategies. First, it provided the middle classes (including small businessmen as well as those employed in sizable industries and organizations) with protection against the one health cost that might be truly burdensome, that is, hospitalization. Families with steady if modest incomes could usually handle a physician's bill on their own, either by postponing payment or negotiating a lower fee. What they could not cope with was the fixed and significant cost of a hospital stay. By insuring against almost all the costs of hospitalization, Blue Cross solved this problem for its subscribers, and in so doing took them out of a potential constituency with a stake in government intervention.

Second, and no less important, Blue Cross energetically set out to persuade the middle classes that national health insurance was not only unnecessary but illegitimate, to render them personally indifferent and intellectually hostile to such schemes. Private insurance, not public programs, represented the American Way.

To understand Blue Cross's successes, one must fully appreciate the magnitude and skillfulness of its campaigns to there enroll subscribers and mold public opinion. Its performance on these fronts was decisive, for without an active and concerned middle-class constituency, advocates were unable to achieve passage of a federal program. Blue Cross helped to secure the definition of health care coverage as a personal and private responsibility. In practical terms, it enabled the middle classes to protect themselves in relatively inexpensive fashion. In ideological terms, it made the case that health insurance not only could be but should be left to the marketplace. Blue Cross self-consciously set out to relieve families and hospitals of the burden of health care costs to the express purpose of reducing the possibility of government intervention. It was not the cunning of history but the cunning of Blue Cross that helps explain the early failure to enact national health insurance.

The history of Blue Cross began in the early 1930s, when many of the country's hospitals were attracted to the idea of a prepaid hospital insurance program, whereby citizens would pay a regular sum in advance and obtain, in return, all the hospital services they required free of charge in the event of illness. In 1929, Baylor University in Dallas, Texas, devised the first of these plans, and over the next 20 years, through the organizational skills of Blue Cross officials, they spread across the country. By 1945, Blue Cross insured 2 million Americans; by 1950, 40 million.[2]

That hospitals were the moving force in devising and implementing these arrangements should not be surprising, for they were having a desperately difficult time in making ends meet. Because of the Depression, contributions to hospitals had fallen off (donors were too strapped to make their gifts), and at the same time, patient fees were down (people were economizing even at the expense of their health). The steady income that would flow from these insurance policies was a godsend, enabling the institutions to survive. Thus from its inception, Blue Cross was a voluntary, not-for-profit organization that was committed to the well-being of hospitals. It was, managerially speaking, in the hospitals' pocket, not merely sympathetic but sub-servient to their interests.

But, that fact acknowledged, the Blue Cross story has other, even more intriguing aspects. It provided real and important financial protection in health care not to a cross section of the American public, but to a very particular subset of it: the middle classes. Specifically, Blue Cross coverage went primarily to employed workers; the preponderance of its membership came from group plans organized through employers. Thus, as one Blue Cross administrator conceded, "The elderly, the unemployed, the chronically ill, and the poor, in large measure [were] left out of the system."[3] By 1947, this bias was altogether apparent. That year, a federal government analysis of Blue Cross enrollments concluded that the plan succeeded most where per capita income was highest. In Baltimore, for example, "the percentage of enrollment varies with economic status—as economic status goes up so does the percentage of the population enrolled." In Rochester, New York, 85% of families with over $5000 a year annual income were enrolled; for those with incomes below $1300, the percentage plummeted to 14.[4] And this inequality of distribution of benefits persisted through the 1950s. As a Brookings Institution study found, there was little room for the unemployed, the disabled, and the elderly in Blue Cross systems.[5]

In effect, to use the language of the insurance world, Blue Cross creamed the population. To keep its reimbursement levels as low as possible, it excluded or made it financially prohibitive for the elderly or the disabled (by definition, high users of medical services) to join its plan. Conversely, it preferred to enroll the employed, who by the very fact of their employment and income, tended to be healthier. Moreover, Blue Cross enrollments coincided perfectly with the ranks of those most likely to vote, those whose preferences and well-being would be paramount in the minds of their political representatives. Thus, to solve the problem of health care for the middle classes was to almost guarantee that national health insurance would not be a politically viable issue.*

---

*Blue Cross also inspired commercial insurance companies to enter the field, so that by 1950, these companies had enrolled another 35 million Americans in their plans. Thus, by 1954, more than 60% of the American population had some type of health insurance, all from marketplace, not public, sources.

Blue Cross did not trust to these demographic and political facts to make certain that government remained outside the health insurance universe. To the contrary, it dispensed a huge number of didactic texts and illustrative images through a wide variety of outlets to accomplish this purpose.

It would not do justice to this output—either in terms of its content or goals—to dismiss it as mere advertising. To be sure, Blue Cross was selling a product, attempting to persuade Americans to buy its insurance policy and enroll in its programs. An organizational self-interest underlay the messages. But that is not the whole of the story, for the product it was selling was unusual, representing not simply a particular solution to a particular problem (as in pharmaceutical advertisements for pain relief), or a highly generalized appeal to an accepted social value (as in life insurance advertisements that emphasize responsibility to family). Rather, from its inception, the Blue Cross effort to sell health insurance was bound up with definitions of what individuals should do for themselves and their families, and what government should do for its citizens.

Analogies to the Blue Cross campaign are not easy to draw, but to grasp its special character it is helpful to imagine an educational system that is privately run, noncompulsory, and relies entirely upon students' fees for support. Were this situation to exist, the schools would have to cajole students and their families to enroll and, in the process, convince them that not only was education worth purchasing but that school was the right place to get it, and a not-for-profit, nongovernment school at that. Such an effort would require an enormous and varied output that would have to address fundamental concerns of individuals, the society, and the state. This was precisely the context within which Blue Cross operated.

In its opening years, Blue Cross had to approach the matter of advertising with great caution, for in health care, advertisements were associated with hucksters and quack remedies; indeed, insofar as physicians' services were concerned, advertising was unethical and illegal. Blue Cross, as a not-for-profit organization with a self-defined mission of service, could not allow itself to be linked with crass commercialism or fraud. Yet somehow it had to persuade subscribers to enroll in its new insurance program, and had to rely upon advertising to attract their attention. As Frank Van Dyk, one of the most energetic and successful Blue Cross administrators, explained in

1934: "The greatest problem encountered in the development of group hospitalization [is] related to the method and policy of promotion. A mere presentation of the benefits listed and emphasis on low cost will not meet the situation. A demand based on a realization of the value of hospital service, its frequency and how this plan meets a community and individual need must be created *before* application can be successfully solicited. This requires training, experience and knowledge of complex problems of hospital operation and public relationship." In other words, Blue Cross faced the same problem as any organization that wished to market a new service: the need to create a demand.

Van Dyk's solution was to launch an extensive advertising campaign. He complained that when group insurance plans were discussed "in hospital circles . . . little concern seems to be expressed regarding the readiness of people to subscribe. One gains the impression that all that is necessary is to put such a plan into operation and that the line of applicants will form on the right." But in fact, attracting subscribers was a far more difficult task. "Even 85 cents a month will buy many loaves of bread for the man with the small income. He must be convinced that he needs this protection and more particularly that he realizes what modern hospital services offer in prevention as well as cure."[6]

Van Dyk brought this central idea to Blue Cross administrators in New York. He proposed (to a 1938 meeting) that "we ought to carry on a state-wide publicity program to make this state hospitalization conscious. The way to do it would be through a planned campaign. This would cost some money, but it would not cost so much that the plans can't well afford to spend it." His advice was heeded, and over the period 1935–1945, Blue Cross administrators, in New York and elsewhere, mastered the art of generating favorable publicity, usually free and always without violating medical norms. They never missed an opportunity to get their message across, and were remarkably adept at calling attention to themselves. The head of Buffalo Blue Cross, for example, arranged to have the local electric company enclose the plan's brochure along with its monthly bill; the arrangement did not offend the Buffalo medical society, despite its opposition "to publicity on the basis that it is not considered [right] for hospitals or doctors to advertise."[7]

Other officials cultivated the art of the press release. Every milestone in Blue Cross history became the occasion for a newspaper story explaining the plan and outlining subscribers' benefits. As one national Blue Cross report explained: "Yearly, quarterly, and six months' enrollment growth stories were released to the Associated Press and United Press, and many newspapers in Plan areas carried these stories." So, too, announcements and photographs of the first subscriber, the one-thousandth subscriber, the five-thousandth subscriber all went out, as did human interest stories about how Blue Cross covered the cost of having triplets or quadruplets, about how it took care of the bills of one family that was unlucky enough to have five members simultaneously enter a hospital, but lucky enough to have all of them insured through Blue Cross. A section devoted to Blue Cross affairs appeared in each issue of *Hospitals*, the official publication of the American Hospital Association, and columns describing Blue Cross activities were often found in such publications as *Hospital Management* and *Modern Hospital*.

Plan administrators went on the radio, with scripts carefully crafted to tell the Blue Cross story and explain, in detail, the roster of benefits. One *Town Meeting of the Air* was devoted to "How to Pay Hospital Bills," and a number of stations aired a special program about "Blue Cross Care for the Farm Family."[8] All the while, Blue Cross distributed to subscribers annual reports that reviewed its activities, and sent separate reports to employers explaining its program. Blue Cross sent a monthly bulletin to its own executives as well as to hospital personnel and trustees, which, it boasted, was also "widely read by civic and employer groups."[9] Periodically, Blue Cross plans would decorate a window in a Main Street department store with a life-size cardboard cutout of a nurse holding a placard: "Are You Protected? Join the Blue Cross Plan." They handed out novelty items like book matches, ran slogan contests (one winner: "Blue Cross Your Bridges before You Come to Them"), filmed movie shorts, gave innumerable talks before professional, business, and Rotary groups, and, finally, beginning with New York in 1943, ran advertisements in newspapers.

Even before exploring the substance of these messages, it should be recognized that they were highly professional products; there was nothing amateurish about Blue Cross campaigns. A "3 Cents a Day" slogan set the trend for short, snappy lines with numbers—as witness the title of an early 1940s Blue Cross movie, *Every Two Seconds* (in reference to the frequency of hospital admissions). A New York City radio version was called "Every Forty Seconds," and a publicity release entitled "On Their Own Two Feet," which was not about the best way to leave a hospital but the American Way in health care.

These campaigns did not entirely escape criticism, not so much at the outset but in the post-1945 period when Blue Cross rates became the subject of controversy. The objections were not about the ethicality of the advertising but about the expenses incurred. The columnist Murray Kempton, writing in 1957 for the union newspaper of the oil, chemical, and atomic workers, chided Blue Cross for behaving like a profit-making monopoly. "Last year," he noted, "Blue Cross spent $2,400,000 for the expense of soliciting subscribers and $465,549.96 for advertising. Those are budgetary items more suitable to a biscuit company."[10] But Blue Cross quickly responded: "Subscribers . . . are entitled to know about the corporation's progress because it is only through sharing of such knowledge that responsible public decisions can be made." Moreover, "Without broad public understanding of the purposes behind Blue Cross it is doubtful whether the public would have responded as it has, and without such continued reporting, it is also doubtful whether Blue Cross could be continued as economically for all who subscribe. . . . The more people Blue Cross enrolls, the better service and lower rates it will be able to offer."[11] Blue Cross was sufficiently confident of the validity of its position to continue to invest heavily in advertising.

To attract subscribers to the Blue Cross plans, the publicity had to accomplish two tasks: one, to make certain that the hospital, more precisely, the voluntary hospital, was defined by the public as the appropriate setting for the treatment of acute illness; the other, to persuade individuals that a group health insurance policy was a sound personal investment. However specific the tasks might appear, they actually raised profound social and political issues. Blue Cross had to set forth both the appropriate method for delivering health care and the appropriate method for paying for it. And because its messages blanketed America, its outlook on these issues played a critical role in shaping middle-class attitudes and practices.

The first proposition that Blue Cross helped to validate was that hospitals were central to the provision of medical care. Although by 1935 this idea was far easier to demonstrate than it would have been a few decades earlier, it was still not self-evident. The transformation of the hospital from almshouse to temple of science was well underway, as witness the fact that hospital use now correlated directly, rather than inversely, with income—the greater the wealth, the more frequent the hospital stay. But the transformation was very recent, and the Blue Cross advertisements made a special effort to present the hospital as the most appropriate setting for delivering care.

To this end, it first taught its audience that the modern hospital, unlike its almshouse predecessor, was comfortable, pleasant, and homelike. The center photograph in one Blue Cross collage of hospital images was of a woman patient in a bathrobe, not hospital gown; an attractive nurse stood at her bedside and adjusted her pillows. On the bedside table there were flowers and an appealing tray of food. In fact, nurses were almost as ubiquitous as physicians in the earliest Blue Cross photographs, their presence creating an ambience of care and concern. When male patients were used in advertisements, they wore hospital gowns—to demonstrate that they were sick, not shirking their responsibilities—and the nurse was holding a thermometer—thereby establishing her professional concern and assuring the viewer that the patient's wife was not neglecting her caretaking duties.

The Blue Cross representations of the hospital included the most technological features of medicine. The patient in the collage was surrounded by images of medical equipment, including the microscope, the X ray, and the paraphernalia for delivering anesthesia. Ubiquitous in Blue Cross presentations was the masked and gowned surgical team. Blue Cross, to be sure, was not alone in celebrating either the caring or the technological aspects of medicine. *Life* magazine photographs, for example, explored both aspects, celebrating the family doctor as well as the latest marvel of research. But the Blue Cross effort was far more systematic and extensive—this was not one photographic story among many but a series of presentations repeated frequently and distributed widely. The hospital was the essential component of good health care. Advanced technologies, sophisticated surgery—these were the hallmarks of modern medicine.

Selling group insurance for hospitalization was a more complicated assignment than promoting the hospital, and to this end, Blue Cross adopted a variety of strategies. In the first instance, the facts of the plan had to be explained and Blue Cross newspaper and radio presentations were heavy on print and information. The New York plan used the services of the advertising firm of J. Walter Thompson, an agency known for being print intensive. The selection was an obvious one for Blue Cross; Thompson's president was deeply interested in health care policy, served on the plan's board of directors, and the agency was among the very first to enroll its employees in the program.

The advertisements had to establish the relative affordability of a Blue Cross plan—the slogan about obtaining coverage for "3 cents a day" did that. And they had to create a felt need for insurance coverage, especially among the cohort that Blue Cross was most eager to attract, the young and the healthy. But how to convince the people who needed it least to invest in a protection plan? Why should a healthy 30-year-old worry about the cost of hospitalization? The Blue Cross answer emphasized the unpredictable character of illness, the sudden and unanticipated onset of disease. One popular advertisement had Blue Cross represented as a helmet protecting the unaware victim against the club of the hospital bill that lay hidden waiting to assail him; the slogan that accompanied the image read: "You never know what jolt is around the corner." In this same spirit, Blue Cross radio scripts recounted the story of one worker who was so confident of his family's good health that he was considering dropping out of the company Blue Cross plan, that is, until he returned home one day to learn that his son has just fallen out of a tree, broken his leg, and would require extensive surgery and hospitalization. By underscoring the unexpected character of health care needs and by emphasizing the notion that illness could strike anyone at any time, Blue Cross set out to create a level of anxiety great enough to attract subscribers without immobilizing or terrorizing them.

Blue Cross messages also stressed how expensive hospital stays were, in a shrewd effort to force potential subscribers to calculate whether they would be able to afford the requisite services. The onus in these advertisements was not on the hospitals—they were not to blame for the high cost, because they were investing in new technologies. Rather, the relevant question was whether the head of the family was fulfilling his responsibility, that is, making certain that his wife and children would be able to obtain the best of medical care in a time of illness.

Not to be able to do so, Blue Cross advertising explained, brought a myriad of penalties. Deferred or delayed hospitalization meant an increased severity of the disease; the patient who was forced to worry about hospital bills recuperated more slowly. Of course, in the background remained the option of using the public, municipal hospital in a time of personal financial emergency, but the Blue Cross rhetoric discouraged this fail-safe mechanism. It could not altogether disparage the services that the public hospital delivered; to do so would be to declare outright that those who used it (that is the poor) were receiving suboptimal treatment, which might then be used to build a case for government-sponsored health insurance. Accordingly, Blue Cross messages took the tack (which would be used again and again in the debates around health care in this country) that neither the rich nor the poor had a problem with health care costs; the one could afford to pay for services, the other could rely upon public facilities. Only its target group, the middle classes, faced a dilemma. They had too much money to qualify for welfare, but not enough money to be certain that they could afford hospital services.

So why not have the middle class use the public system to meet an unanticipated calamity? The Blue Cross answer suggested, more subtly than explicitly, that the public system provided too minimal a level of comfort. Blue Cross gave semiprivate, two patients to a room, accommodations; here, not in a 12- or 16-bed ward, one received "the best of attention." In fact, Blue Cross advertisements actually never showed the second bed. To judge by the images, every subscriber had a private room filled with flowers. Surely at a time of illness, one would want one's wife to enjoy middle-class standards of privacy.

Not content that such appeals made the case strongly enough, Blue Cross vigorously and unabashedly labeled the public hospital a public charity, with all innuendoes intended. It declared outright that respectable citizens should be responsible for their own care, not having recourse to the dole. The story line of the Blue Cross program, "Every 40 Seconds," exemplified the approach. The dialogue was between father and son about the ill mother who was reluctant to seek medical help:

> Paul: Why doesn't Mommy let you call the doctor?
> Father: We'll talk about it later, son.
> Paul: Well, gee, she looks so sick.
> Father: . . . She'll be all right, so don't worry . . . .
> Paul: Look, Dad—if Mommy let you call the doctor and he would send her to the hospital and they gave her good care there and lots of good medicine and the nurses did everything for her and she'd be nice and comfortable and wouldn't have any pain, she'd get well real fast, wouldn't she?
> Father: Yes, I guess she would.
> Paul: Well, gee, we just can't sit here doing nothing.
> Father: Son, you're not old enough to talk about things like this—but mother doesn't want a doctor or a hospital because she's worried about the money. . . . And you see, Paul, we're still paying back the money we borrowed when you were ill.

The program then cut to an interview with Louis Pink, head of New York Blue Cross, who explained that "there are many instances of this kind, where people are too proud to accept free medical and hospital care. . . . Apparently Paul's mother is too proud to accept free care. She is accustomed to making her own way—even though she has to fight for it. It is the people in the middle income group who often find it most difficult to secure adequate medical and hospital care. It is sometimes said that the very poor and the rich—if there are any rich left—get the best medical care." And Pink then went on to explain, in full detail, the Blue Cross plan.[12]

The same point was made more succinctly when Frank Van Dyk, attempting to persuade a group of labor leaders to join Blue Cross, insisted that the worker in need of hospitalization who lacked personal resources ought not to be forced to accept "service in wards at part-charity rates." He should not be compelled to establish himself "as a recipient of charity."[13] To be dependent upon state services was clearly an unacceptable alternative. "The average man with the average income," explained yet another Blue Cross story, "has pride. He is not looking for charity; he is not looking for ward care. He wants the best of attention for himself and his family. . . .

Yet out of his savings, he is very seldom prepared to meet unexpected sickness or accident expenses."[14] In effect, to use the municipal hospital system was to be stigmatized as poor and dependent, incapable of standing on one's own two feet. Like the dole, the public hospital was not the American Way.[15]

To the purpose of unambiguously distinguishing Blue Cross from the dole, messages to would-be subscribers stressed not only the trappings of comfort and the importance and satisfaction of paying one's own way but the fact that voluntary hospitals would treat subscribers kindly and courteously, just like paying customers even though no money changed hands. Since Blue Cross was one of the first organizations involved in delivering a service without the open and tangible exchange of cash, it was all the more vital for it to differentiate itself from the public sector and assure its subscribers that neither their reputations nor their treatment would suffer. Thus Frank Van Dyk eagerly shared with a reporter from a woman's magazine letters from satisfied subscribers that illustrated this point: "Members are admitted to hospitals—welcomed you might say—with no more red tape or questioning than those who come in independently. And they are treated just as well as if they were handing out cash." The illustrations that accompanied an article entitled "The Luxury of Illness," showed a woman patient in a hospital bed that resembled a hotel room, and as befit an era when rates of occupancy were low and concern over the cost of a stay were not uppermost in every administrator's mind, the patient informed a friend: "I'm getting a two week rest and some very expensive treatments and it's costing me only eighty-four cents. Come on over and *don't* forget the cigarettes."[16]

To reinforce this message, photographs of Blue Cross subscribers were immediately recognizable as middle class and "respectable." The male models, for example, always wore suits and ties. Through the 1950s, New York Blue Cross rarely used a black model in its advertisements, in another effort to make certain that no one confused its members with those who went to public hospitals. As we have seen, to judge by enrollments over the period 1935–1945, it clearly succeeded in the task.

All of these themes were part of a much larger agenda, the Blue Cross determination to define the respective spheres of government and private initiative in health care. Its aim, succinctly put, was to justify a policy preference for the private over the public sector, for individual subscriptions over government subsidy. As vital as it was for Blue Cross to attract and retain middle-class subscribers, it was no less central to its mission to prevent the federal government from entering the field of health insurance, at least insofar as the middle classes were concerned. Not only for reasons of self-interest—its own and its affiliated hospitals—but for reasons of political philosophy, Blue Cross devoted substantial energy to representing its goals as the embodiment of the American Way.

Against the backdrop of the report of the Committee on the Costs of Medical Care in 1933, which raised the prospect but did not explicitly endorse greater governmental involvement in health care, Blue Cross presented itself as the appropriate alternative to federal intervention in health care.[17] Rufus Rorem, the organization's first head, was indefatigable in making known that supporting Blue Cross was the best way to forestall a compulsory national health insurance system, and state administrators, such as Homer Wickenden, joined him in spreading this message: "The group hospitalization plan, because it . . . avoids any semblance of politics, leaves medical matters in medical hands, hospital matters in hospital hands. And because it is potentially popular, it may be the principal factor in avoiding a system of compulsory health insurance in this country."[18] Another state official put the argument still more concisely: if Blue Cross succeeds, "it should eliminate the demand for compulsory health insurance and stop the reintroduction of vicious sociological bills into the state legislature year after year."[19] When, in 1940, Franklin Roosevelt, in a speech dedicating the new National Institutes of Health facilities at Bethesda, seemed to rule out the "socialization" of medicine, Dr. S. S. Goldwater, then the president of the New York Blue Cross, hailed the message as a "green light" to the organization and lectured labor leaders "to promote non-profit prepayment plans . . . to meet the needs of working people for assured hospital care in all emergencies." Socialized medicine, he was certain, was "staggering in cost, difficult to administer and doubtful as to the kind of service it would provide." Concluded Goldwater: "Our hospitals can function as free and independent institutions only as long as they can function free from government control. . . . Employer and employee groups [should] now get together in a serious effort to make socialized medicine unnecessary for any regularly employed worker."[20]

The issue of national health insurance remained prominent during the war years, mostly because of the introduction in 1943 of the Wagner-Murray-Dingell bill, a cradle-to-grave national social insurance bill modeled upon programs in Great Britain.[21] The opposition of Blue Cross leaders to the bill took the form of an advertising campaign that wrapped itself in the flag and linked the slogan of "be prepared" to the home front battle against disease. Using war metaphors to buttress its concept of the American Way, the texts proclaimed: "The ability of American men and women to 'stand on their own two feet' when faced with emergencies has long been part of our national tradition," and enrollment in Blue Cross belonged to this tradition.[22] Blue Cross also sought to counter the Wagner bill by linking an aroused spirit of patriotism to voluntarism: "The Blue Cross Plans are a distinctly American institution, a unique combination of individual initiative and social responsibility. They perform a public service without public compulsion."[23] The plans exemplified "the American spirit of neighborliness and self-help [which] solves the difficult and important problem of personal and national health."[24] All these propositions led inexorably to the conclusion: "Private enterprise in voluntarily providing hospital care within the reach of everyone is solving the public health problem in the real democratic way. The continued growth of the Blue Cross Movement might well be considered the best insurance against the need of governmental provision for such protection."[25]

In the immediate postwar period, when congressional initiatives made the prospect of national health insurance loom still larger, Blue Cross repeated these principles in every possible forum. When one unhappy subscriber complained that hikes in Blue Cross rates were bringing the country closer to socialized medicine, Louis Pink defended the increase and observed: "The only answer to socialized medicine would be the growth of Blue Cross and other cooperative plans. Socialized medicine would cost a great deal more and would encourage much more abuse than the voluntary plans."[26] Pink also expounded this lesson to radio audiences: "Some people seem to think that all we have to do is put some kind of compulsory

law on the books . . . but that would be putting the cart before the horse. . . .
Whether we shall need a compulsory law or not depends largely upon the
ability of voluntary organizations to make good medical care available."[27]
And other Blue Cross leaders repeated this message. The front page of the
national *Blue Cross Bulletin* of May–June 1948 featured a photograph of
Paul Hawley, its chief executive officer, with the caption: "I am convinced
that the provision of health care under the government would be the most
extravagant experiment the taxpayer has yet been forced to support. He would
pay not alone in money, but in his own health and in the health of those
dependent upon him."[28]

Many Blue Cross executives as well as hospital administrators and trustees deemed the campaign against national health insurance to be at the core
of the organization's mission. One Michigan hospital director, who spear-
headed an extensive Blue Cross publicity drive in 1948, boasted that government officials and political leaders already realized "that they must chart
their course of political action in the field of health care in accordance with
the tides of Blue Cross. Of necessity, then, we are committed to a program
of public relations. . . . We must make sure that our activities are so well
known to the public that the planners of Health Utopia will never have use
for the timetables they are preparing so diligently." These advocates of "political medicine" insisted that voluntary plans cannot perform as well as
government in meeting health care needs. Hence the number one objective must be to "convince the public that Blue Cross . . . is performing a
function which offsets any necessity for government control of health service. In practice and in theory, we in Blue Cross know this to be the truth —
let us say it as plainly as that."

Taking his own advice to heart, this Michigan executive organized a
media campaign in which "public education messages" on the theme of
"The Way of Democracy" appeared in 100 state newspapers and magazines.
These presentations defined the American Way in terms of voluntary group
action, and the texts were accompanied by illustrations of Lincoln "because
we felt that he . . . was the prototype of the American way of life," and of a
town meeting hall "being the symbol of democracy." They were dispatched
to every Michigan state legislator, its congressmen and senators in Washington, and to all the members of the Senate Committee on Labor and

Public Welfare. The publicity generated hundreds of requests for information on membership (although this was not part of a subscription drive) and a congratulatory letter from Senator Arthur Vandenberg: "I believe this is a splendid development in your Blue Cross program. You have 'hidden your light under a bushel' far too long. . . . This is the practical way to check-mate all-out 'socialized medicine.'"[29]

There can be no exaggerating the intensity with which many Blue Cross officials and supporters pursued the drive to block national health insurance. National officers urged their state counterparts to devote more resources to advertising in order to influence congressional legislation. "The story," Rufus Rorem declared, "must make it clear that Blue Cross protection is more comprehensive and economical than the alternatives of . . . a government plan." Abraham Oseroff, vice president and secretary of Blue Cross in Pittsburgh, explained that Blue Cross membership drives were nothing other than "the test case of America's desire for continued self-government. . . . They have become the first line of defense for continuation of the American way of life."[30] And as Roy Larson of *Time* magazine told a meeting of New York Blue Cross officials: "What advertising did in the war for the Government and the armed forces in the interest of the country, it can do now in peace for such a uniquely American way of securing the health and welfare of our peoples through the Blue Cross plan."[31]

On one level, none of these actions is surprising. Blue Cross was an extraordinarily successful example of voluntarism, and from Tocqueville on, the American way of life has been linked to strong associational activities. Given the conflicts over national health insurance, Blue Cross would inevitably attract both to its management ranks and to its cadre of public supporters persons who were convinced of the dangers of a state-run health program. And making Blue Cross the test case for democracy did prompt the organization not only to conduct a vigorous negative campaign to thwart socialized medicine but to make some effort to expand its own roster of subscribers to demonstrate that the private sector was equal to the task of insurance.

But Blue Cross was never ready to open its membership ranks widely. In these years, the plans generally limited their enrollments to the employed—either through formal membership criteria or by keeping the cost of individual subscriptions high. The Blue Cross rhetoric at times suggested that it was *the* answer to the needs of *all* Americans, and some plans did experiment with procedures that reached beyond the usual categories for new subscribers. But for the most part, the indigent and the aged who had not previously been part of a Blue Cross plan or who could not afford the rates were outside the network.

Blue Cross was caught in something of a paradox, for as little as it wanted government involvement in a national health care scheme, so it insisted that Blue Cross should not be subsidizing charity care in voluntary hospitals. More frequently in private but occasionally in public as well, Blue Cross officials advocated government subsidy of the indigent even as they insisted that voluntarism was completely sufficient to the task of health insurance. Oseroff, for example, was indignant about "the folly of expecting plan subscribers to bear a share of the cost of free patients," and many others expressed this sentiment.[32] But for obvious reasons, the organization could not pursue the point too vigorously. Rather, its public presentation obfuscated the critical division between the employed and the indigent, posing the question of health care delivery as though the voluntary sector could satisfy all needs, and omitting consideration of those at the bottom of the economic ladder. Blue Cross did not take as its responsibility exposing the limitations of public hospitals or the number of citizens, young and old, who were unable to join a voluntary health program for lack of personal resources. These considerations might be thought to lie outside its purview, except for the fact that Blue Cross framed its mission as a test case for democracy. But it was a test case of a biased sort, casting the debate on health care exclusively in terms of how to serve middle-class Americans, with scant attention to the fate of others.

Beginning in the post–World War II period, Blue Cross used its advertising to fulfill one more objective: to justify the rising costs of health care, particularly hospital care, and in this way to defend its increases in subscriber rates. Its strategy was to link mounting expenses to medical breakthroughs, in the process making itself one of the most avid and effective promoters of high technology medicine. In the hands of Blue Cross, the American Way in medicine became a paean not only to voluntarism but to new machines and novel procedures. Just as it discouraged government intervention it encouraged a mystique of the machine — at once promoting and reflecting the essence of American values in health care.

As a program that provided subscribers with services rather than cash indemnity (as commercial insurers did), Blue Cross rates were more quickly affected by increases in hospital expenses. But almost every time it went to raise its rates, Blue Cross faced not only a barrage of negative newspaper publicity and subscriber complaints but extensive hearings before state insurance commissions.

The concern about subscriber fees first surfaced in 1947–48. Heretofore, the costs of hospitalization were a fact that Blue Cross could, and did, cite as the very reason why people should join its plan. But the issue was not yet acute, for everyone conceded that postwar inflation was affecting many aspects of American society, and hospitals were only one more case in point. Louis Pink explained in annual reports to subscribers that "the world has probably never been more unsettled. . . . Solutions are being sought on problems of world security, prices, an unstable economy. . . . It follows that in the hospital and medical field we must have some problems too." Hospitals required adequate compensation in a period of continued inflation, and Blue Cross rates were tied to average hospital costs and federal indices of inflation. What Pink emphasized most was that Blue Cross would not cut its benefits and adopt a scheme of partial indemnity, which would put more of a fiscal burden on the subscribers (and, left unsaid, hospitals as well). He even invoked the decision not to cut benefits as one more example of the superiority of Blue Cross to commercial insurers; they were "leaving their members to foot the balance due the hospital."[33]

But as inflation cooled, hospital costs continued to climb, and in the 1950s, Blue Cross faced a series of hostile inquiries. At times, it responded by trying to duck responsibility, claiming that "Blue Cross has no authority over hospital costs." It also promised to institute "a few common-sense limitations on the coverage provided," or to audit hospital services to make certain they were "necessary for the patient's proper treatment." In one New York State rate hearing, a commissioner and several speakers suggested that Blue Cross undertake to control or (more euphemistically) supervise and regulate hospital costs and expenditures. But plan officials demurred, insisting that "there is not any power in Blue Cross, directly or indirectly, to run the hospitals, or, through the hospitals, to practice medicine and conduct, control or dictate the services therein." Moreover, "Hospital costs cannot and should not be frozen. Hospital services cannot and should not be controlled or dictated by Blue Cross or by the Superintendent of Insurance," for such a policy would be tantamount to socialized and state-run medicine.[34]

Blue Cross did not rely exclusively on these defensive and not altogether persuasive responses. The major justification for rising health care costs, as framed by the advertising agency of J. Walter Thompson, was to link them to new advances in life-saving medical technologies. Mounting medical costs became the inevitable by-product of medical progress. Thus, in its post-1950s advertising campaigns, Blue Cross relied even more heavily on images of medical machinery. Its representations of the new technologies appeared below such headlines as: "How to Stop a Heart . . . *Without* Skipping a Beat"; "How They Freeze Brain Cells to Check Parkinson's Disease." According to Blue Cross, the glories of medicine rested in sophisticated technologies and daring procedures, even if they happened to increase health care costs.

The minutes of the J. Walter Thompson planning meetings reveal how self-consciously this campaign was crafted. The Blue Cross "problem," as the account executives defined it, was that the public thought its rates were too high, which generated widespread dissatisfaction and an attrition in membership. "The public," the Thompson executives believed, "thought of Blue Cross as a means of getting their hospital bills paid. There is not a general understanding of the fact that the helping dollars Blue Cross pays provides income which put hospitals in the financial position of being able to advance to new frontiers and have on hand the latest life saving equipment."[35]

Starting from this premise, Thompson designed a series of advertisements to foster "an understanding of why higher rates have been necessary." The campaign would "clarify the facts about increased hospital costs, and attempt to establish a more favorable atmosphere for the necessary Blue Cross rate increase and to do it well in advance."[36] In essence, it would celebrate the capabilities of the new medical technologies, and attribute to them the responsibility for higher costs. Thus, one message about artificial hearts read: "How Machines That Work Like You Are Battling Our Number One Killer"; the accompanying text explained that "Blue Cross Dollars Help to Pay for the Miracle Machines." So, too, according to the agency's 1963 advertisements: "Today's hospitals are better staffed and better equipped than ever, including complex, expensive and often quickly obsolete machines."[37] In the end, Blue Cross found itself rationalizing spiraling expenditures as the unavoidable consequence of medical innovation. In the world according to these advertisements, citizens gratefully paid ever increasing dues, recognizing that saving lives through technology was an expensive business.

Just how original and consequential the Blue Cross messages were is apparent from a comparison of its advertisements with commercial medical insurance companies, particularly the Metropolitan Life Insurance Company. Metropolitan Life came to health insurance in an effort to extend the reach of its own enterprise by providing its life insurance subscribers with yet another package to select. In 1952, it introduced personal hospital and surgical policies for individuals and families which provided cash indemnities according to a preset schedule. But Met Life, more diversified in its policies than Blue Cross, did not have the same unyielding commitment to private health care programs; nor was it so tied to the support of voluntary hospitals. Accordingly, its promotional campaigns took a very different tack, not contravening the Blue Cross message on the American Way, but advocating, in a far less political fashion, preventive health care. Both organizations, quite obviously, stood to benefit when subscribers stayed fit and used fewer hospital services. But Met Life, more systematically than Blue Cross, attempted to encourage good health care habits and behavior.

Met Life campaigns did not feature the marvels of high tech medicine or surgical teams. Rather, they urged people to see their physician, more precisely their general practitioner, at the earliest sign of illness. "What is the right thing, the *safest* thing to do when trouble comes? *Get Your Advice from a Physician!*" The illustration that accompanied the text, "How Innocent Is a 'Stomach-Ache'?" depicted a physician making a house call; he was standing at the bedside, holding a thermometer and talking to the mother. The text went on to urge "prompt medical attention" to stomach pains, warning that deaths from appendicitis were three to four times higher among those who ignored the symptom. Still another advertisement depicted two toddlers traipsing through the snow, one saying to the other: "Just like Mommie says—if you catch a cold and get a fever, go to bed and she'll call our doctor to come see you." However unlikely that two children would carry on such a conversation, Metropolitan Life continued to instruct readers on "Why every family should have a family doctor," explaining that in no other way would it obtain all "the benefits of preventive medicine," and cautioning that a doctor's black bag "is not a 'do-it-yourself' kit."

Even the few advertisements in which Metropolitan Life did pay attention to the hospital (generally during National Hospital Week) were notably different from Blue Cross campaigns. The illustration for "What If Your Hospital Closed its Doors Today?" labeled the low-slung building "Community Hospital" (no tertiary medical center for Metropolitan Life), and the illustrative cases were not of a heart that stopped beating but of a child who swallowed a poison. The appeal to support hospitals (in 1963) had a photograph of a closed hospital door with a "No Visitors" sign, and the text explained how the patient needed "peace and quiet," without so much as a mention of medical technology. There was no excitement, no glamour, and no reason to believe that hospitals represented anything so special that one would want to enroll with Blue Cross rather than Metropolitan Life.

The comparison with Metropolitan Life makes clear how unique and focused the Blue Cross message was. For some 30 years it produced a surfeit of texts and images that sought to persuade Americans to insure themselves against health care needs, to do so on a voluntary basis, and to accept increasing costs as the corollary of medical advances. Although Blue Cross was not alone in advocating any of these positions and one can never be certain of the degree to which its campaigns created or reflected popular values, nevertheless the success of its membership drives and the data available from public opinion polls indicate a considerable impact.

Beginning in the 1940s and continuing thereafter, poll data consistently revealed a widespread public appreciation of the need for health care coverage, for some type of protection for the individual citizen against the costs of illness. "Consumer Attitudes toward Blue Cross and Blue Shield," a study prepared for J. Walter Thompson in 1961, found that "health insurance [is perceived as] a must. . . . Health insurance has become increasingly sensible and necessary in people's thinking and their attitudes toward available plans and sources is very positive . . . [They] contribute broadly to security and peace of mind." Indeed, "the public is sympathetic and knowing in general ways about the fact that doctors, hospitals and drug companies have had to keep pace with rising costs and increase their rates accordingly."[38]

The public also seemed to agree with the proposition that twentieth-century medicine was high technology medicine to which they should have unlimited access. As the 1961 survey reported: "Medically people are inclined to take as much as they can get. . . . They feel that they are, in this rich and progressive country, entitled to have the techniques of modern medicine available to everyone at any time."[39] There was some ambiguity about whether health insurance should be left to the private sector. "They are not much concerned whether or not medicine is socialized to some extent, although they feel very sure that the AMA and many doctors individually probably would not like it. But they feel that medicine has become so complicated, so specialized and so expensive that industry and government should work with the individual to carry the medical load." These wavering sentiments, however, did not become a stimulus to national health insurance. For as we shall see, in the hierarchy of values, access to medical technology for the middle classes came first. So long as the private sector was able to deliver heroic medicine, the middle classes had little incentive to bring government into health care.

2 The Iron Lung and Democratic Medicine

The first encounter of Americans with life-saving medical technologies was the iron lung, a clumsy but often effective machine that was capable of rescuing polio victims from imminent death. Invented in 1928 by Philip Drinker and widely distributed immediately thereafter, the iron lung became the occasion for Americans to express and absorb the values that would continue to influence national attitudes and practices decades later. Around this device, Americans formulated their initial ideas about allocating scarce medical resources. It is here that we find the origins of the ethic that life-saving technologies had to be available to everyone, that the prospect of benefits, however slim, outweighed the costs, however substantial. And it is here that the message Blue Cross so energetically spread received compelling reinforcement: that the private sector was fully capable of meeting the challenges which the distribution of scarce and powerful medical resources presented. Through private initiatives, not government programs, this country could escape making hard choices about allocation. To the question of who lives, who dies, the answer could well be, everyone lives.

The iron lung was the first assemblage of parts (to adapt Webster's dictionary language) that transmitted energy and motion from one segment to another for the purpose of performing a life-saving task. Like many other medical devices, it was born of an immediate clinical necessity. In some patients, the poliomyelitis virus paralyzed the intercostal muscles of the diaphragm, impeding the automatic ability to breathe. Before the invention of the iron lung, those suffering from acute and short-term muscular paralysis could be kept alive by having someone manually squeeze and release an airbag until the intercostal muscles regained functioning. But such extraordinary assistance could be sustained only for a day or two, and hence, patients with long-term paralysis inevitably died.

In 1928, building on some earlier but cruder devices, Philip Drinker, an engineer appointed to both the Department of Applied Physiology at the Harvard Medical School and the Department of Industrial Hygiene at the Harvard School of Public Health, designed the iron lung. He was at least as interested in aiding victims of industrial accidents as of polio. To build his prototype, Drinker received a grant from the Consolidated Gas and Electric Companies of New York, whose chief concern was with asphyxiation due to accidents; its rescue squads were regularly called upon to administer artificial respiration to victims of carbon monoxide poisoning, drowning, and drug overdoses.[1] "In order to prove satisfactory," Drinker explained, "such an apparatus must be capable of working steadily over a long period of time; it must be adaptable to individuals of various ages and sizes; it must be so constructed that the rate and depth of respiration can be controlled; last, and most important, it must be capable of producing adequate artificial respiration without discomfort or harm." His device accomplished all of that. The patient was placed in a tank 66 inches long, 22 inches in diameter, large enough to hold a man 6 foot, 4 inches tall or a small child. A rubber collar was adjusted around the neck—to make the machine airtight—and then "by means of electrically driven blowers, alternate positive and negative pressures are applied to the air within the tank." When the pressure in the tank was negative, the diaphragm contracted and the patient inhaled; when the pressure turned positive, the diaphragm expanded and the patient exhaled. The rhythm could be maintained indefinitely.[2]

Drinker and his team of physiologists, which included his brother, Cecil, and Louis Shaw, tried out the machine first on cats, and then on Drinker himself and on Shaw (in the best tradition of medical experimentation). The first patient to use Drinker's iron lung was an eight-year-old girl admitted to Boston's Children's Hospital with fever, aches, and pains. Physicians quickly diagnosed her case as polio, noting paralysis along some sections of her intercostal muscles. Realizing that her respiratory functioning would soon cease, they called Drinker, who came over with his machine. Before putting her in the machine, as one of the physicians, James Wilson, later recalled, they pondered the ethics of their action, fearful that patients might have to live in the iron lung for the rest of their lives. "There was no experience to guide us," Wilson noted, "but there was a feeling that since some muscle power did come back in the arms and legs, it might come back in the respiratory muscles and, therefore, the attempt was justified."[3] For five days, the device sustained her breathing. On the sixth day she died, not from muscular paralysis but from infection; an autopsy revealed that neither lung had suffered any damage. Accordingly, concluded Drinker, the machine was useful and appropriate for patients who required sustained artificial respiration.

No sooner did Drinker announce his breakthrough than the iron lung went into production and distribution. Once the prototype proved effective, Consolidated Gas and Electric donated a machine to Bellevue Hospital's accident ward, and in the spring of 1929, the device saved the life of a young woman who had inadvertently taken a drug overdose. A few months later, in September 1929, a senior at Harvard contracted polio and was rushed to Peter Bent Brigham hospital in severe respiratory distress. Physicians placed him in the iron lung and within several weeks he recovered completely. He graduated from Harvard, and as Drinker happily reported, "now walks, almost unaided, goes to work down town, drives a car, and what is more important, has been in good health constantly since his dismissal from the hospital."[4]

Drinker assigned the patent for the machine to the Warren E. Collins Company of Boston, and for the next five years it was the exclusive manufacturer. The new technology was quickly dispersed, not through government intervention but by private philanthropic efforts. Community organizations and local charities raised the $2000 to $3000 necessary to purchase the machine. By June 1930, New York City had 12 iron lungs (courtesy of the Consolidated Gas Company), Boston had 6, and Philadelphia, 2. By November 1931, 150 respirators were found in hospitals all over the country. The New London, Connecticut, hospital received its Drinker respirator "through the generosity of Mrs. Edward S. Harkness"; the Glen Cove, Long Island, hospital, through the fund-raising drive of the ladies auxiliary organization; and New York's Willard Parker Hospital, through a grant from the Jeremiah Milbank Fund.[5]

The initial eagerness to equip local hospitals with the iron lung was not as naive and innocent a response as might be supposed. From the very start, there was a professional and popular recognition that this technology was not unambiguously advantageous, that it carried risks as well as benefits. Although the appearance of a life-saving device was bound to generate exaggerated claims and overenthusiastic endorsements, the iron lung also met with a surprising degree of caution, even skepticism, about the efficacy of the intervention. The case of the Harvard undergraduate made the device seem remarkable; the iron lung would save lives and return healthy and fully functioning citizens to the community. But as a number of physicians and patients soon discovered, the reality was far more complicated, to the point that some of them wondered whether the device did more harm than good.

Part of the wariness resulted from the fact that the iron lung was over-used, with patients placed inside it even when their paralysis was untreatable by the machine. The device was useful against only one form of polio, inter-costal paralysis, but not against a second form, bulbar polio. Bulbar polio irreversibly damaged the nerve cells in the breathing center of the brain and these nerves would not regenerate over time. The iron lung could take over for intercostal muscle, which in the majority of cases would return to func-tioning; however, once the brain centers were damaged, there was nothing that the iron lung could do. Despite the fact that this distinction was well understood, physicians confronted with a dying and gasping patient often had recourse to the respirator.[6] Recognizing that the intervention was fu-tile, but hoping against hope, they tried it anyway—and in the process built up an association, both statistical and anecdotal, between high levels of mortality and the use of the iron lung.

Also tempering the enthusiasm for the machine as well as diminishing its effectiveness was the very complicated issue of timing the intervention: at what point in the patients' illness should they go on the iron lung? Was it when they first experienced breathing difficulties, or when their symptoms worsened, or when their distress was acute? Answers varied from hospital to hospital, depending in part on how readily available an iron lung was and in part on how familiar the physician was with the mechanism and the dis-ease. The greater the distance that the patient had to travel and the less the sophistication of the physician, the greater the likelihood that patients would be sicker upon entering the iron lung, and the greater the likelihood that they would not enjoy a complete cure.

These considerations, together with high rates of mortality from infec-tion in a preantibiotic era, drastically reduced the successful outcomes of iron lung treatment. In the summer of 1931, for example, physicians in New York City reported that of the 88 polio patients in four city hospitals who went on the Drinker respirator, 53 (or 60%) died in the hospital. Of the remaining 35 patients who had been discharged from the hospital and were able to breathe without artificial aids, 16 had soon died, mostly from pneumonia. "These additional deaths," noted the report, "bring the final mortality of the respirator-treated cases to the appalling figure of 78.4 percent."[7] Results were no better in 1932. In Brooklyn, of the 65 patients with intercostal paralysis put on an iron lung, 49 died and 16 survived. "Of those who are still living," noted the report, "practically all have almost complete paralysis."[8] In Westchester, one hospital used the Drinker machine in 16 cases; but only four of the patients lived and three of them suffered continuing paralysis of upper and lower extremities. Reviewing this dismal record, concluded the report, "brings up a question of the ultimate value of the machine for poliomyelitis."[9]

Other physicians were more enthusiastic about the efficacy of the intervention, although their outcomes were only marginally better. In Boston, of the 30 patients who went on the iron lung between 1930 and 1931, 17 died; "hospital mortality," reported the physicians, "has been reduced by more than one-third through the use of the respirator." Their paper, however, said nothing about the quality of life of the survivors and glossed over the fact that the majority of iron lung patients had not survived.[10] So, too, an international survey of treatment outcomes, conducted by the British Medical Research Council in 1938, reported 84 survivors of a total of 234 patients in the iron lung; of the 84, 38% were dead within four years, 20 percent had no or only slight paralysis, and the rest (42%) were invalids or bedridden. To put the findings most concisely and soberly, only 17 of the 234 people treated with the iron lung returned to a fully normal life.[11]

The public also had its reservations about the machine, prompted not only by the statistics but by the intrinsic character of the intervention. As so often happens, a new medical technology enters popular awareness through a particular case, and Frederic Snite was to the iron lung what Barney Clark would later become to the artificial heart. If anything, Snite's was the more sensational story. The son of a wealthy financier, he was touring China with his parents in the spring of 1936; on arrival in Peking, he felt ill, complaining of dizziness, fatigue, and aches. Although everyone presumed that he had a bad cold, the symptoms grew progressively worse to the point that one arm became paralyzed. The family called in doctors from the Rockefeller Foundation–supported Peking Union Medical College Hospital, who examined him and diagnosed his case as polio. Snite entered the hospital, but his condition rapidly deteriorated until he was about to lose all respiratory functioning. By an amazing coincidence, the hospital had an iron lung—the only one in all of China—secured through the largess of the foundation. Until that moment, it had been used only for patients suffering an overdose of opium. Snite became its first polio patient, beginning his dependence on artificial respiratory machines that lasted until his death in 1954.[12]

Snite remained in the Peking Medical College Hospital for 14 months—a local bank contributed an air-conditioning unit to counter the heat—and, in the process, became a media novelty. His fame, newspapers reported, spread to the point where "most of literate China recognized him as "The Man in the Iron Lung." The American press covered Snite's saga in great detail, outdoing itself in describing his trip back to the States. Dispatches turned it into "the most outstanding medical odyssey of all time." Reporters stood by at every stop, rail and sea, to watch how he, and his machine, were transferred from one generator to another. Even after his return home, the press still paid attention to the story, letting the public know, for example, that Snite had switched from an iron lung to a smaller device that fit over the chest.

But along with the celebration of Snite's victory over death came a no less acute sense of dread and revulsion about the personal ordeal that such treatment imposed. The most popular designations for the new technology suggested strength, durability, and awesome power, truly an iron lung. Other descriptors, such as "hope chest," carried the connotation of rescue and aid. Yet alongside these favorable terms came darker images of a casket, a prison cell, a sense of entrapment and entombment. Some newspaper stories described Snite as a prisoner in a "casket-like steel box," confined to his "iron cage." They said the same of another similarly afflicted patient, Gene Roehling: "His life hangs by the wheezing of a leaky iron lung. He can't move a muscle below his neck, pain is perpetual and a power failure a deadly emergency. Here's the story he tells from his one-man prison." A life spent trapped in a cylindrical tube apparently was no life at all.[13]

However profound these misgivings, they did not undermine a national commitment to make the machines everywhere available. Another set of values intervened to override the doubts. Within ten years of the invention and production of the iron lung, hospitals in the United States purchased and installed some 700 of them. Why this determination? Why the insistence on obtaining an iron lung when the mortality and morbidity rates associated with it appeared so discouraging? Even as the strengths and limitations of the technology were better appreciated, the drive to make the machine available to all who might possibly need it accelerated. To understand the roots of this ambition, and how firmly it became part of American values toward medical technologies, we must turn to the most remarkable of American philanthropic organizations, the National Foundation for Infantile Paralysis.

The National Foundation for Infantile Paralysis (NFIP) was the most successful private voluntary organization ever to enter the field of health care. Founded in 1937 by President Franklin Roosevelt, and directed by Basil O'Connor, a one-time Wall Street attorney, it raised $622 million in its first 12 years of operation and had more volunteer workers in its ranks than any other such organization, before or since. The NFIP supported research and, still more heavily, the delivery of clinical services. Perhaps best remembered for funding the research that culminated in the discovery of the first polio vaccine, the organization devoted the bulk of its considerable resources to insuring that no patient with polio was deprived of necessary medical services because of economic hardship. To this end, the NFIP defined economic hardship very liberally: it was prepared to underwrite the support of care to polio patients whenever medical expenses were so large that they might force a family to lower its standard of living. It also defined medical services very broadly, ready to reimburse patients for the expenses of rehabilitation and to reimburse hospitals for recruiting professional staff and for purchasing equipment. It was this sense of commitment that brought the NFIP to the iron lung.[14]

Its program was devised with considerable forethought and planning. In January 1939, the NFIP asked two New York physicians to review the subject of respirators. They reported back that the respirators functioned extremely well (not often needing repairs), and "frequently they have been the direct means of saving a life."[15] Since the machines were expensive and were usually required on an emergency basis (when an epidemic suddenly struck a community), the consultants recommended that the NFIP purchase 50 iron lungs, place them at regional centers around the country, and arrange for their loan as communities needed them.

The NFIP moved carefully on the recommendation, commissioning a fuller survey in 1941 by James Wilson, a pediatrician and leading researcher in polio at the Children's Hospital of Michigan. Wilson informed the NFIP that some 400 to 500 polio patients a year were treated in iron lungs, almost one-third of them children under the age of 10, and 70% under the age of 20. Wilson complained, however, that a large number of these patients (over 60%), were suffering from bulbar polio and probably did not benefit at all from the intervention; worse yet, over a quarter of those who could benefit from the technology went on the machine too late. (Some of the reason for the delay, Wilson believed, was "because of the frightening appearance and the disturbance" that the use of this "big, coffin-like apparatus . . . causes in a hospital.") Finally, Wilson cautioned the NFIP that "we have no good data, nor can we probably expect to get any, regarding the social value of the patients 'saved' with the use of the respirator." With a survival rate of 80% of patients with intercostal paralysis, clearly the machine was keeping a significant number of people alive. But there was now no way of knowing whether the life saved was worth living, whether the disability was so grave, or the dependence on the machine so total, that it cast doubt on the wisdom of the intervention. "Certainly we can say," concluded Wilson, "that a considerable number become competent individuals."[16]

The NFIP published Wilson's report, and the response to it revealed just how controversial the use of the iron lung continued to be. Morris Fishbein, editor of the *Journal of the American Medical Association*, summarized its findings and then commented: "Although Wilson's report does not make the definite statement, it is clear that the use of respirators for poliomyelitis is often disappointing. This device certainly does not approximate the high expectations for saving lives or treatment originally predicted."[17]

Wilson, despite his own and others' misgivings, still urged the NFIP to use its resources to make the machine everywhere available. It was not an easy decision for him to reach—or for the foundation. The decisive arguments came in a letter from Wilson to Basil O'Connor in June 1941. It opened with a most extraordinary concession, really an admission: "I could wish, as I believe you do, that as far as poliomyelitis goes the respirator had not been invented. Throughout the country there are several dozens of horribly paralyzed patients, who seem quite useless and are a tremendous burden and expense to someone. Without the respirator these patients would have died and adjustments to their loss long since made." In fact, these unfortunate patients were so overwhelming in their demands, and in their plight, that "most doctors and hospitals dislike having the respirator around since the possession of a machine may lead to a responsibility which will become very troublesome and expensive."

Nevertheless, Wilson continued, "the only realistic attitude is to accept the fact that the respirator is here, that it will save life . . . and . . . in our present state of social development there can be no question whatever of not using a respirator for a patient that needs it." Despite the fact that he and many other physicians shared an unremittingly negative view of life with a disability, and that they typically approached the issue of handicaps almost exclusively from the perspective of the care giver, not the disabled person, they were unwilling to allow the technology to remain in short supply. Again, reservations about democratizing the technology, however well based they seemed to those who held them, were cast aside.

Accordingly, Wilson laid out the plan that the NFIP soon implemented, in effect enlarging on the earlier, 1939, recommendations. The NFIP would immediately purchase a number of respirators (in this way "the price of respirators could be greatly lowered") and distribute them to centers around the country. Wilson recognized that "plans regarding the number of respirators to be needed must be made more or less arbitrarily and that it is not practical or wise to try to place within each community enough equipment to wholly meet any possible emergency that might arise within that community."[18] Hence, the regional facilities were to lend out the machines when epidemics exhausted a community's own resources.[19]

How should Wilson's and the NFIP's commitment to making the machine everywhere available be understood? Why did they come down on the side of national distribution, rather than adopting some kind of implicit rationing? The answers are of special importance, for they provide an invaluable context for understanding the origins of American attitudes toward the allocation of scarce and life-saving medical technologies.

The NFIP decision exerted an immediate and powerful influence not simply on polio patients but on thousands of people around the country, in effect teaching them the importance of making medical machines available. The NFIP was composed of 3000 to 4000 thousand local chapters, staffed by at least 100,000 volunteers. At the same time, its campaigns for funds, in which the iron lung was a very prominent feature, spread its message to ordinary citizens everywhere. No less important, the messages themselves and what the NFIP actually accomplished were perceived by the public as relevant for polio in particular and for medicine, health care, and democratic obligations more generally.

The role of the NFIP is better appreciated by briefly noting how different the British experience was. In 1938, Lord Nuffield made a generous offer to pay the entire cost of the "Both" breathing machine for any hospital that would use it well. (The Both machine was made of wood, not iron, and hence the British use of the term *breathing machine* as opposed to iron lung. The wooden machine, of course, was less expensive than the Drinker machine, and may not have been as effective.) The Nuffield gift resolved the question of access to this medical technology for the British.[20] However, because it was a charitable act by a single individual, not the starting point of a public campaign, the issue was taken off the public agenda and divorced from ongoing social or political considerations. Here may be one more reason why in England access to medical technology was not associated with democratic processes or outcomes.

Thus we are brought back to the importance of the presumptions that underlay the NFIP commitment. Precisely why was it so determined to provide widespread access to technology? The first part of the answer rests with the physicians' influence over the organization. They brought to its mission a medical mind-set, older than some contemporary analysts may appreciate, that emphasizes the successes, however limited, and disregards the failures, however more commonplace. In this mind-set, an ability to save even one life trumps all other considerations.

The first reactions of Boston's Dr. Reginald Fitz to the iron lung testify to the power of this perspective. He had, it seems, been "rather doubtful about the machine at first. It looked cumbersome, it was noisy, and it seemed more like a torture chamber than anything else." But then "one boy that I saw get well in it entirely convinced me as to the practical value of this method of giving artificial respiration." For Fitz, and for many other physicians, the single success outweighed all the failures. And so Fitz concluded: to cope with "epidemics of infantile paralysis in the future, hospitals treating such cases should be equipped with the respirator. One life saved is worth a lot, and it is comforting, at least, to have something in the line of rational therapy to offer those cases of respiratory failure which heretofore were doomed."[21]

The physicians who consulted with the NFIP shared this outlook, ready to promote a commitment to making the iron lung available to save some lives even at the price of many failures. Admittedly, physicians' ambivalence about the machine was keen, and some doctors were reluctant to put patients into a coffinlike apparatus; in the abstract, as Wilson observed, many a physician "would rather have his patient die than his life saved in a respirator only to become a hopeless cripple."[22] But in actual practice, when the patient's symptoms worsened and breathing became more difficult, physicians used the machine, and did so even for cases of bulbar polio, where it was almost certainly useless. Confronting a dying patient, doctors would do something, anything, rather than just stand there, or even give comfort. Although they might later regret having preserved a life that was to be spent confined within a tomb, they acted no differently the next crisis round.

In this same spirit, physicians were convinced that their pro-iron lung bias, whatever the consequences for the patient's eventual quality of life, was shared by the general public. Wilson did note that he had "encountered a few lay people, philosophically inclined," whom he believed "would be willing not to use a respirator on a member of their family if I had talked convincingly enough about dire future possibilities of crippling." But with most people, and "particularly with doctors whose own children have a suspicion of respiratory paralysis, the urge for the immediate use, or at least availability of a machine, is tremendous." In other words, the decision became personalized, framed in terms of using it to save one's own child and, thus, by ethical necessity, to save another's child. (We will return shortly to the importance of the fact that children were the typical patients for the machine.) And it was not only medical ethics but medical legal liabilities that were at stake. "No death from this disease," Wilson declared, "can occur without the question of the use of the respirator being brought up." Should a patient die in a hospital which did not have an iron lung, "the implication that the hospital has not been properly equipped frequently arises."

Moreover, a kind of medical optimism made everyone more comfortable with the allocation decision. Wilson, as well as other infantile paralysis specialists, was confident that time would bring improvements in physicians' use of the iron lung. They believed that most general practitioners waited too long before getting patients on the machine, thereby reducing its effectiveness and increasing the likelihood of bad outcomes, specifically, patients becoming respirator-dependent. The crux of the problem, as they defined it, was an insufficient supply of iron lungs. Many physicians still had to send a patient some distance to use one, thereby severing their own relationship to the patient, putting the family to great inconvenience, and placing the patient at significant risk during the journey. Furthermore, general practitioners and pediatricians would not learn how to use the machine properly so long as it was not readily available and in close proximity. Unfamiliarity with the iron lung perpetuated outmoded attitudes (about its coffinlike appearance) and practices. However, poor practices and negative stereotypes could not be permitted to impede the spread of the benefits of the intervention. Abundance would prevent the abuses that scarcity promoted. Multiply the machines and doctors would use them appropriately. These were the precepts that guided medical technology in a democratic society.

Second, and perhaps even more important, the NFIP as an organization was particularly receptive to this credo. Guaranteeing full access to a new medical technology fit perfectly with its own sense of mission and purpose. As befit a body whose origins and continued functioning were so intimately connected to an American president, and one whose rhetoric and programs were clearly tied to the well-being of all citizens, regardless of social class, the NFIP almost instinctively brought a democratic ethos to questions of access to medical technologies. Not surprisingly, it defined the death of any patient because an iron lung was unavailable as its own institutional failure. "To attack the problem of smooth, inexpensive equipment supply," observed one NFIP executive, "it may be well to consider the responsibilities that, we of the N.F.I.P., have assumed as our duty to polio patients. Those responsibilities can be summed up by our wish to provide every patient the wherewithal to reduce his suffering and increase his possible chances to recover or improve. . . . In my opinion every lack of the needed facilities whether it is for a single patient, or for a thousand cases — creates an emergency condition."[23]

Adopting this proposition, and making it fundamental to its fund-raising appeals, the NFIP could not—and would not—tolerate any shortfall between promise and performance. "We must at all costs," insisted George Voss, the national epidemic coordinator, "avoid the possibility that the National Foundation might be criticized because we failed to either offer or provide respirators in any locality where they are needed."[24] A death that might have been prevented through an iron lung was thus defined not as evidence of the dreadfulness of a virus but of the inadequacies of the NFIP, and perhaps even a reflection on its founder, FDR.

Third, the NFIP stance and the impact of its message on American attitudes was at once reflected and reinforced by the epidemiological characteristics of polio. For one thing, most polio victims were children and teenagers; in 1940, for example, at least two-thirds of patients reported with polio were younger than nine years old. Although in the post–World War II period, the percentages of those over nine would rise, polio continued to be perceived as a kid's disease.[25] Accordingly, a commitment to distributing the technology had all the more appeal. The philanthropic tradition of serving the well-being of children became a critical component of attitudes toward medical technologies. This was, after all, *infantile* paralysis.

The NFIP's many publications assured that the youthfulness and innocence of the victims of polio would receive great prominence. Children always occupied center stage. In one poster campaign, run under the caption, "Join the March of Dimes," an attractive six-year-old girl with braces on her legs, stands next to an iron lung, with the implicit message that she owes her life to the machine. In a widely distributed NFIP pamphlet describing how one community, with the NFIP's assistance, handled a polio epidemic, several pages are devoted to photographs of "Some of the Children your Dimes and Dollars Helped." Kenneth, the youngest patient, seven months old, lies in his bassinet, clad in his diaper, smiling up at the camera; Jerry, a winsome two-year-old, stands holding onto the bars of his crib. There was a head shot of Judy, an adorable three-year-old, and a photograph of Logene and Minnie, two teenagers, lying in adjoining beds, a partially completed jigsaw puzzle between them. These pictures implicitly declare that to deny any one of these children a life-saving intervention was not simply wrong but unforgivable. Both to the foundation and to the public which so generously supported it, it became apparent that the prospect of victory, not the grimness of defeat, had to dictate policy toward medical technology.

Fourth, were the ages of the patients not reason enough to democratize access to the machine, considerations of social class were relevant as well. From the very start, allocating scarce resources was an issue that was framed in terms of the needs of the middle classes. Polio, oddly enough, was predominantly, although not exclusively, a middle-class disease. It disproportionately struck children raised in hygienic, uncrowded, and, epidemiologically speaking, protected environments; in 1936, for example, the polio rate per 100,000 of the population was 7.2 in the case of whites and only 3.3 among blacks.[26] (Children from lower class, urban backgrounds were more likely to be exposed to the virus at a young age and therefore built up immunities to it.) In this sense, polio was a disease probably found more often among the haves than the have-nots—even apart from the extraordinary symbol of an aristocratic president as one of its victims. The class bias meant, among other things, that donations to the NFIP were not charitable gifts to help "them," but a self-interested effort to protect "us." Polio, at least after the 1920s, was not defined as an affliction bred by neglect, poor diet, inadequate housing, or immoral conduct; it was not akin to tuberculosis (the disease of the ghetto), let alone cirrhosis (the disease of the alcoholics). And, of course, the NFIP made this point prominent in its literature: "Infantile paralysis is not primarily a disease of the slums, the malnourished or the underprivileged," declared its 1942 pamphlet, "Doctor . . .

What Can I Do?" "Rather, it often seems to pick out the healthy and the active for its victims."[27]

In this way, the NFIP's commitment to guaranteeing access to the iron lung built on and called attention to the respectability and blamelessness of polio patients. The prevailing vision was of devoted parents rushing their stricken child to a local hospital, hovering over the doctor as he made his examination, and pleading with him to do all possible to save the child's life. The idea that a physician might have to say that no machine was available was unthinkable. Middle-class children were not going to die in America because iron lungs were in short supply.

One final element framed both NFIP and public conceptions about guaranteeing access to a new medical technology. The iron lungs were to be distributed through a network of volunteers; the task was to be achieved by private, philanthropic means, not governmental programs. To demonstrate just how feasible this goal was, and to make the effort altogether intrinsic to the meaning of a democratic society, the NFIP itself as well as the press frequently drew on military metaphors, particularly on the "home front" experience. By chance, the complicated issues that surrounded the national distribution of iron lungs assumed an acute importance during and immediately after World War II. Thus, the theme of the self-styled campaign was to get the iron lung to the front—this at a time when Americans excelled at organizing military campaigns and took enormous pride in them.

The NFIP was particularly adept at invoking the metaphor so as to garner financial support. Its pamphlet, "Miracle at Hickory" read like a description of an eminently successful invasion, a kind of D-day against disease, this one staffed by volunteers, not conscripts. Hickory, North Carolina, population 5000, in the foothills of the Blue Ridge Mountains, did not even have a local hospital when polio struck in epidemic proportions in the summer of 1944. The community rapidly mobilized its forces, and in a matter of days, volunteers transformed a summer camp for underprivileged children into a 150-bed hospital. The effort represented a remarkable tribute to the spirit and efficacy of doing good on a personal level. "Workmen bringing their own tools came and asked to be allowed to work. . . . Housewives cooked food in their own kitchens and brought it to the hospital until a kitchen and dining room could be built and staffed. Business and professional men and women dropped their accustomed activities to lend hands unaccustomed to manual labor to whatever tasks were necessary. . . . Units of the State Guard voluntarily spent their Sundays working around the hospital. . . . Governor Broughton paroled thirty-two women prisoners to ease the load of hospital housework." At the same time, "skilled polio fighters, supplies and equipment were being dispatched by the National Foundation" and doctors were being "rushed to the scene." Should anyone miss the military analogy, the pamphlet included a photograph of "the wife of a general in the invasion forces" nursing a child in the hospital, and prominent in the scene was a newspaper headline: "Allies Advance in Twin Drives in Normandy." On the opposite page of the pamphlet, another photograph showed a group of men unloading an iron lung, looking ever so much like a group of gunners readying a torpedo.[28]

The evocation of volunteers in a quasi-military campaign on behalf of polio patients continued to frame the NFIP coverage of iron lungs into the post–World War II period. The trip that Bernard Green made from West Haverstraw, New York, to the Children's Hospital in Baltimore (as presented in another NFIP photographic essay) had the aura of troop maneuvers. The opening picture was of fellow patients standing outside the 45-foot ambulance, looking just like the families that gathered outside the army buses that took their boys off to boot camp. The bus shortly encountered snow (photo of police shoveling out a clearing), and then later, a flat tire (photo of townspeople helping to change it). The closing shot showed the iron lung being wheeled into the hospital, 48 hours later, the mission complete.

The presentations unambiguously conveyed the message that just as Americans had joined together to secure democracy against the Axis powers, just as they had manufactured and transported war equipment to bring victory on the battlefront, so they were now duty bound to unite against polio and ship to the front a very different, but no less vital, type of equipment. Americans had successfully made armaments, now they would make iron lungs; the drive and talent harnessed to equip soldiers would go to equipping doctors. To do anything less was to be cowardly, even un-American. A spirit of patriotism joined to voluntarism permeated medicine, furnishing still another incentive to maximize the distribution of the new technology.

Working from these premises, the NFIP put into place a most remarkable, and in the field of health care, unprecedented system to realize this goal. In the process, it taught Americans that the private sector was perfectly capable of translating a commitment to open access to medical technology into practice. The NFIP purchased iron lungs, transported them, repaired them, reshipped them, and kept accurate tallies, like a quartermaster corps. The organization even had a mobile emergency field unit, what it called a "hospital on wheels," to transfer iron lung patients from one care facility to another. The record for the greatest distance covered went to a 15-year-old girl, a kind of local Snite, who underwent a transfer of some 900 miles, traveling from Florence, Alabama, to the Children's Hospital in Baltimore.[29]

The NFIP appreciated that such efforts would create still more demand and that the burdens of care would spiral upward, fostering a dynamic that Americans in the 1990s would come to know very well. "We have found," observed one NFIP administrator, "means of keeping patients with respiratory involvements alive for longer periods, increasing the need for respirators. As we continue to progress, more patients will be placed in respirators for rest periods. In fact we are utilizing respirators more and more each year." Thus, in 1948, the NFIP transferred 141 machines among communities. Nineteen forty-nine posed even heavier demands because some 1948 patients were continuing to use their machines, creating a need for the NFIP to obtain still more respirators. So the NFIP purchased an additional 144 iron lungs and transferred 803 of them from place to place; it tripled its express charges and quadrupled its repair bills.[30] It was a record year, an extraordinary accomplishment, and compelling testimony to how voluntarism and the private sector could meet desperate needs.

These efforts gave each iron lung an odyssey of its own. Machine S#41 was purchased August 6, 1941 by the NFIP, and was immediately shipped to Jasper, Alabama; after use there, it was repaired and stored until being sent on August 3, 1942 to Nashville, Tennessee, and then on August 27, on to Morgantown, North Carolina. In November 1944, it went to Brooklyn, New York, and later, in August 1945, to Hempstead, Long Island; in August 1946, it was sent to Forth Worth, where it became part of the San Antonio pool.[31] Between 1941 and 1946, Machine #753, went first to Philadelphia, then to Hickory, North Carolina, then to Nashville and Lexington, Tennessee, then to Milton, West Virginia, back to Boston for repairs, and then on to Pittsfield, Massachusetts.

To be sure, there were headaches and even dirty dealing. Coordinating its own equipment with the respirators owned by other health care facilities brought the NFIP a variety of administrative difficulties. One of its officials discovered that in emergency situations hospitals with iron lungs "are willing to transfer only the old ones." "I have seen these machines," the official noted, "and feel strongly that they should not be borrowed . . . [unless] it is impossible to get along without them." Again, as befit its organizational credo, the NFIP official insisted: "Because of the public relations connected with the transfer and use of respirators and because of their life saving nature, we cannot afford to leave ourselves open to criticism by furnishing any but the best. For that reason we must obtain machines that are dependable."

Even such complications did not deflect the NFIP from its goals. It worked well with the Emerson Company and made it central to the NFIP's pooling and storage efforts. "The company takes a personal interest in all polio equipment, effects necessary repairs, and has worked around the clock to keep the equipment moving. . . . All concerned know that we had no worries about the condition of the equipment when sent to hospitals for use."[32] This kind of alliance allowed the NFIP to live up to its promises, make the iron lung accessible to those in need, and, in the process, demonstrate the effectiveness of volunteer efforts.

One final lesson emerged from the NFIP accomplishments and the iron lung story: not to worry excessively about risks and costs when benefits from medical technologies could be obtained. As the number of patients using the iron lung multiplied, so, inevitably, did the number of patients who had difficulty coming off the machine and breathing on their own. The incidence of complications was low—less than 5% of all users—and most often resolved within a matter of months, not years or decades. Nevertheless, the symbolic importance of patients totally dependent upon the machine was considerable, and so were the demands that they placed on health care providers.

To judge by the frequency of patient and press accounts of the problem, the public was at once simultaneously fascinated and repelled by the idea of entombment in the machine. In fact, a dread of a horror movie scene come to life might have provoked a revulsion against the machine, one that was potentially severe enough to curtail its use and undercut a commitment to diffusing medical technologies. But this was not the message that went out, not from the NFIP and not from those who actually suffered this sad fate. The accounts of life trapped inside an iron lung, or more accurately the accounts that were published, invariably adopted a positive frame. The narratives had a heroic tone, which, if anything, heightened the commitment to distributing the machine.

The titles of the iron lung narratives did feed a morbid fascination. Jim Marugg called his book *Beyond Endurance*, and Leonard Alexander, his, *The Iron Cradle*. But the substance of these autobiographies was far more hopeful and encouraging. "Blessed be the things which cannot be endured," proclaimed Marugg. "It is when I am farthest down that I lift myself highest up." After Frederick Snite's death, his attendant for 17 years, Leonard Hawkins, recounted the story of *The Man in the Iron Lung*, and the book's dedication conveyed the same moral: "To the polio patients of the world, whose courage I have tried to reflect here."

Hawkins's account described in rich detail the good times that Snite had—how he loved playing bridge and watching horse racing, how he displayed a keen sense of humor, introducing himself at a March of Dimes benefit as "the boiler kid." For several years, Snite was able to spend part of the day on a smaller, portable chest respirator, and he married and fathered three children. (Hawkins, as befit an English-born attendant, gave no details about the marriage or Snite's sexual life.) Only occasionally did some of the agonies that Snite endured emerge. A religious Catholic, he went to Lourdes, "to ask God to give me the strength to live in this tank for the rest of my life." But the overriding lesson that both Snite and his biographer steadfastly sought to convey was inspirational: Snite going on a tour of veterans hospitals to tell World War II disabled soldiers to keep the faith; Snite informing the press that illness was a maturing experience: "Your sense of values changes. Religion and my family have become the important things in life, and that is as it should be."[33] Life in the iron lung was a trial, but only one of the many trials that life presented.

Jim Marugg wrapped his maxims of uplift in athletic metaphors. He recounted how he entered the iron lung suffering from paralysis and high fever, and how the terror of being "caged" almost led him to abandon hope. Apparently he overheard his doctor telling a nurse: "Well, I've done all I can. I guess the guy's given up. He's quit fighting. . . . Better call his wife." Even so, reported Marugg, the physician pleaded with him to do battle: "You know what it is to call up the last ounce of strength it takes to win a race. This is a race. You can make it if you try. . . . You just can't quit." Marugg met the challenge, in the process coming to appreciate the simple, and best, things of life. The experience "taught me how good a thing it is to be able to go to work in the morning, how fine to be able to go home in the evening—how wonderful to go to sleep at night." Life took on a new meaning. One learns to endure.[34]

Lawrence Alexander's autobiography is far more revealing of the despair that could overwhelm the iron lung patient. He unflinchingly reported his deep ambivalence toward the machine, at once eager to be rid of it but at the same time attached to it on both a physiological and psychological level. When he first went on the machine, he feared he would never come off. "What kind of life would it then be?" he asked himself. "Where would I find the strength or courage to keep on with it?" But after a few days, when the device relieved him of the need to struggle for every breath, "the metal respirator assumed an almost animate personality and became a symbol of protection and security. The idea of leaving it [to breathe on one's own] would always make our hearts beat a little faster. . . . We were incomplete embryos in a metal womb," tied to the iron lung through an umbilical cord. After spending a few hours outside breathing, painfully and haltingly, returning to it "was like running back to your mother's skirts, to a safety and security that you can trust completely." His dependence, and regression, first generated anger and then depression: "How much of a life would it be if I went on like this, unable to move, unable to help myself in any way, immobilized forever in this metal coffin? Was that any better than death? . . . To spend my future in this steel womb was no life at all, no life I wanted."

But Alexander ultimately made peace with his disability. After two years of physical rehabilitation, he was completely weaned from the respirator and, wheelchair-bound, was able to return home. As he reviewed his experience, he was most intent on demonstrating his spiritual progress. He discovered service and helping others, doing good for his neighbors and community. His triumph, as he summarized it, was not only over polio but narcissism.[35]

The iron lung narratives are fascinating for what they affirm: those who underwent the ordeal survived. However terrifying the experience of being trapped in the machine, those who faced it endured, coming out better at the end. To be sure, the narratives of illness are a genre that require this type of ending; to justify the act of writing and publishing, the patient must end on a life-affirming note.[36] But whatever necessary construction underlay the tales, the message was unambiguous. Better life through technology than no life at all.

The narratives are also fascinating for what they omit. There are no episodes in which a patient asks to withdraw from the machine, or tries to withdraw from an iron lung. Neither the narrators nor anyone they encounter seek to terminate treatment. Perhaps in the real world such requests did occur, and it is conceivable that some iron lunger persuaded his doctor to stop treatment. But if such events took place, they were kept secret and were never discussed openly. Hence, the messages that the public heard contained only success stories, triumphs of spirit over body, of mind over disability.

This united front gave no opening for a discussion about limiting the use of a life-saving technology because of a patient's refusal to accept it. And absent this consideration, it was all the more difficult to begin a dialogue about limiting the use of a life-saving technology both from an individual and from a societal perspective. The only questions that had to be addressed were practical and administrative: how best to meet the needs of those who needed the machine, and how to cope with the problems of those unable to come off the machine.

Having already noted how well the NFIP managed the first assignment, it is not surprising to learn that it also did quite well by the second. It experimented with new medical and rehabilitative techniques to wean iron lung–dependent patients; at the same time, it made the chronic care of these patients integral to its programs. Rather than abandon them to state or municipal long-term care facilities, as other agencies and providers did with the chronic mentally ill or with those suffering from an "incurable" disease, the NFIP maintained its responsibility. As a result, the fact that expanding access to a technology inevitably increases the burdens of care did not come back to haunt the NFIP, or, for that matter, subvert its original commitment. The burdens that came with democratizing access to machines appeared manageable, even without government intervention.

Thus, in November 1950, the NFIP reported that 583 patients were dependent upon the iron lung (defined as those remaining on respirators for longer than one month). The large numbers reflected an increased incidence of polio (1949 and 1950 had been epidemic years), a rise in the number of older patients contracting polio, and higher survival rates for respirator cases because of improvements in the equipment, better trained personnel, and the powerful effects of newly discovered antibiotics. Respiratory infections that once proved fatal were now easily contained.[37] These numbers — and the expense of caring for them — did prompt a policy review at the NFIP. It turned out that iron lung–dependent patients were treated at 135 different hospitals. So, both to provide more expert care and to reduce costs, the NFIP established regional respirator centers. The centers were charged to promote research into how best to manage respirator therapy, acute and chronic; to administer training programs in respirator management for medical personnel; and to treat the most difficult chronic cases. As Basil O'Connor explained in announcing the new strategy: "Iron lung cases are the most tragic of all polio cases. If we can wean even a few of them from their mechanical breathing devices, it will be worthwhile."[38]

The NFIP soon had respirator centers operating in Los Angeles, Houston, Ann Arbor, Boston, and Buffalo. Over 1952 and 1953, these centers accepted some 300 machine-dependent patients, who on average had already been hospitalized for nine months. Within a year, the several centers were able to discharge 80% of the patients home; almost half of them were completely weaned from the machines, and the remainder were able to use smaller aids (like the chest devices), some or all of the time.[39] The NFIP was never able to get all respirator-dependent patients into its own centers, and it complained that because of the inadequacies of treatment elsewhere, the "patients do not progress and tend to remain for very long periods or indefinitely in hospitals. More tragic than death itself perhaps is the fate of many of these patients, who survive the acute attack, and are destined to remain dependent upon the tank respirator because of lack of adequate care."[40] In other words, the NFIP acknowledged the nightmare cases, but put the blame on the institutions, not the machines. So long as experts managed the technology, society had nothing to fear from medical progress.

Nor did anyone have to be concerned about the financial costs of care. Discussions about the nationwide distribution of iron lungs devoted some, but only some, attention to the economics of making such a commitment; most important, and without exception, the findings minimized the impact. The consensus was aptly summed up by one speaker at the First International Poliomyelitis Conference, in 1948: "Although our efforts ought not to be restricted by considerations of cost, the public, who ultimately pays the bill, is entitled to get value for money."[41] The issue, as framed by this first encounter with life-saving medical technology, was not price but quality.

Not that the sums were trivial. For the hospital, the cost of purchasing an iron lung rose from $1350 (in 1939) to $2000 to $3000 (over the 1940s), owing to the wartime increase in the price of raw materials, especially chromium and aluminum. For the families, the expenses might have been ruinous. As Chester Keefer, fresh from his service in supervising wartime research and the distribution of penicillin, observed: "The disease is often long-term in nature and requires large sums of money to pay the costs of illness and rehabilitation. Poliomyelitis often places families in serious financial straits and the expenses of doing everything possible and necessary in order to prevent death, limit disability and rehabilitate victims of the disease are more than most families can afford." Patient bills averaged $1000, distributed among the hospital (41%), nursing (19%) and physicians (19%).[42]

But costs turned out to be a minor consideration to the larger society and the particular families, in large measure due to the fund-raising capabilities of the NFIP and its readiness to support families generously. As the superintendent of the Buffalo Children's Hospital informed his colleagues in their trade publication *Hospitals* in what reads like a paean of praise both to technology and voluntarism: "The general hospital should not hesitate, from a financial viewpoint, to admit infantile paralysis cases. If no person or agency is responsible for the payment of hospital care, the local chapter of the national foundation will assume the responsibility. . . . Hospital administrators will find . . . the foundation eager to cooperate in making possible adequate medical care under proper hospital conditions for the infantile paralysis patient." And this commitment included necessary purchases as well: "Equipment must be obtained . . . respirators, suction machines, treatment table. . . . A hospital faces not only a terrific physical hardship, but a financial one, when it is required to take care of an epidemic. Again, the national foundation has relieved the situation. There is hardly a reason for the general hospital to deny admission to polio patients."[43]

The foundation was not extravagant or careless in its responses, but it did meet its obligations fully. When funds ran low during the 1949 epidemic, the NFIP appealed to the public for additional donations and asked physicians (through the *Journal of the American Medical Association*) to reduce fees "without prejudice to the patient" by trying to be more sparing with hospitalization, less dependent upon specialists, and more receptive to home care. All the while, the NFIP carefully worked out polio fee schedules with state medical associations, making certain that when the foundation assumed responsibility for a family's medical bills, the outlays would be predictable without provoking the ire of organized medicine. "By no means," declared foundation officials, did the NFIP "wish to interfere with the *physician-patient relationship.*"

Accordingly, state and local chapters were instructed to contact an attending physician and ask him (not demand from him) whether he would accept the NFIP fee schedule; the chapters also left it to the physician to select the hospital for treatment, obviating the fear that the NFIP might make exclusive contracts with particular hospitals in return for reduced rates. In this same spirit, the NFIP reimbursed families only for ward beds, not for semiprivate or private rooms, making certain not to undercut private insurance coverage. Finally, the fee schedule that it set was eminently fair—the attending doctor, for example, received $75 for the first month in an uncomplicated case, $100 for a complicated case, and thereafter, $5 a home visit in the city, and $10 in the country.[44] In no way was this particular and exceptional venture in voluntarism going to undercut others—or taint itself by incurring the opposition of the medical profession.

To be sure, the NFIP had some help in its mission. There were available relatively inexpensive insurance policies that covered polio alone, and the federal government, under the Social Security Act, did give states funds for the care of needy crippled children. But these measures did not have nearly the impact of the NFIP program, or its publicity.

In sum, the NFIP succeeded in taking the issue of reimbursement for polio out of medical or national politics, and in so doing, gave yet more distinctive attributes to this first encounter with life-saving medical technology. It made a life-saving medical technology available everywhere and to everyone, regardless of region or socioeconomic class, and in disregard of less than optimal medical outcomes. At the same time, it helped eliminate considerations of cost as a determinative consideration. In all these ways it inaugurated a mind-set about medical technologies, democratic obligations, and cost considerations that persisted for decades to come.

3 | Medicare for the Middle Class

From the New Deal until the mid-1960s, health insurance remained, at its core, a private responsibility. Exactly as Blue Cross and an expanding number of commercial insurers, like Metropolitan Life, had hoped, and in accord with the demonstrated abilities of voluntary organizations like the National Foundation for Infantile Paralysis, there seemed little need to bring government into the health care field. Not just ideology but performance confirmed the adequacy of the marketplace. It was not only that Americans shared a persistent distrust of government, but that in their own lives and in their everyday experiences, they felt no need to change the system. Periodically, legislation would be introduced to expand government health programs, but whether the initiative came from Congress, as in the 1943 Wagner-Murray-Dingell bill, or from the White House, as in the case of Harry Truman, it suffered defeat. The United States remained almost alone among industrialized countries in not providing national health insurance.

In this framework, the passage of Medicare in 1965 outwardly represented a new departure in American health policy. For the first time, the federal government guaranteed that all citizens over the age of 65 would have access to hospital services. Repudiating allegations that it was socializing medicine, Congress enacted and Lyndon Johnson signed a bill that provided the funding to enable the elderly to forgo reliance upon private health insurance and enter hospitals at little expense to themselves.

Although proponents expressed the belief, at the time privately and later more publicly, that its passage was to represent the first step on the road to national health insurance, in fact, Medicare turned out to be a dead end. It was not unreasonable to anticipate that once the government provided health insurance to those over 65 it would eventually come to serve those under 65, but the expectation proved wrong. In the aftermath of the 1965 legislation, only the elderly (and the very poor, through the very differently administered and far less liberal program of Medicaid) experienced a shift in health care costs from the marketplace to the government. Everyone else still had to turn to the private sector to buy protection or otherwise pay their own medical bills. For the great majority of the country's citizens, Medicare made no difference.

Most commentators have accepted the premise that Medicare was intended to be the opening wedge that would bring national health insurance to the United States, and, accordingly, they have treated those who promoted and enacted the bill very generously. Whatever the causes of later failures, the proponents of Medicare seemingly had nothing to do with them. But these interpretations do not look hard enough, or skeptically enough, at the central ideas that accompanied the passage of Medicare or even its operating principles. As paradoxical as it may appear, the messages that went out from Medicare's most ardent supporters and the internal design of the program buttressed and reinforced the idea that health care belonged first and foremost to the private sector, that health insurance was to be purchased in the marketplace. The elderly were carved out as an exception—but an exception that would allow the traditional mechanisms to continue to enjoy their dominance. Why this should have been so is well worth analyzing, for the agitation on behalf of Medicare demonstrates the staying power of the historical record that we have been exploring, the disadvantages of promoting a policy built upon exceptionalism, and, finally, the implications of framing policy strictly in terms of the needs of the middle classes.[1]

The reasons for government inaction in health care have engaged a number of scholars, and the well-crafted arguments of two of them, James Morone and Paul Starr, go a long way to clarifying, in the broadest sense of the term, the political dynamics that were responsible. Morone's frame for understanding American health policy in general and the failure of national health insurance in particular, as put forward in *The Democratic Wish*, focuses on popular definitions of the proper role of the state, the lines that citizens drew around acceptable or not acceptable governmental programs.[2] Morone acknowledges the critical role that the unbending hostility of the American Medical Association to national health insurance played in the process. But while others characterize AMA rhetoric as bombastic, comical, or even hysterical, Morone insists that it was highly effective precisely because it tapped widely shared assumptions about the appropriate relationship between governmental authority, professional capacity, and professional autonomy. By the terms of this consensus, the government's duty was to build up professional capacity without infringing on professional autonomy—and so long as the medical profession defined national health insurance as an infringement on its autonomy, such a policy would not be enacted. These conceptions permitted government to fund hospital construction (organized medicine had no problem with the implementation of the Hill-Burton Act in the period immediately after World War II). And they certainly allowed government to endow the research establishment (as witness the extraordinary growth of the National Institutes of Health over these same years). But they did not permit interventions that would challenge or subvert professional autonomy as delineated by most physicians and enunciated by the AMA.

Paul Starr, in *The Social Transformation of American Medicine*, also invokes conceptions of state authority to explain the outcomes of health policy.[3] Alert to the markedly different course of national health insurance in European countries, he posits that where a spirit of liberalism and a commitment to the inviolability of private property interests in relation to the state were strongest, movements for social insurance made the least headway. Thus Bismarck's Germany could accomplish what Franklin Roosevelt's or Harry Truman's United States could not. Put another way, the fact that socialism never put down strong roots in this country, the absence here of a socialist tradition or threat, obviated the need for more conservative forces to strengthen their own parties and, at the same time, buttress the social order through welfare measures.

Starr is more ready than Morone to credit the raw political power of the AMA, but he also reminds us that the AMA found allies not only among corporations but labor unions. Union leaders preferred to obtain health care benefits for their members through contract negotiation, not through government largess — even if that meant, or precisely because that meant, that nonunion members would go without benefits.

Other scholars have added vital points to the analysis. Theda Skocpol focuses on both the limited administrative mechanisms available to the state and the public perception of their weak capabilities to explain why health care remained a private enterprise.[4] Lawrence Jacobs, at least in part, attributes the reluctance to bring in government to peculiar American ideas about health care itself, the depreciation of the value of primary care as against what the iron lung story exemplifies so well, the romance with higher technology and hospital-based medicine.

Their particular emphases notwithstanding, these judgments on the political process and definitions of the proper role of government point to a social fact of enormous importance: that well into the 1960s, the middle classes experienced no acute need for federal intervention in health care. They negotiated their (usually small) bills with their private physicians and insofar as hospital coverage was concerned, those who were gainfully employed either purchased their own insurance protection or received it as part of their job benefits package. The rolls of Blue Cross expanded and labor unions became more adept at including health care coverage in their new contracts. Thus, there was no solid middle class constituency moving any of the critical features of health care from the private to the public sector.

Then, in 1965, after several years of defeats, Congress unexpectedly did undertake to provide all Americans over the age of 65 with health care coverage. The campaign for Medicare began in the late 1950s. Reformers such as Wilbur Cohen presumed that a program that covered only the elderly, and was limited to paying their hospital bills, would garner greater support from the public and from Congress; its more narrow reach (both in terms of who it covered and what it covered) would seem less threatening, and might help bring it in under the mantle of the very popular and widely accepted government Social Security program.

From the European perspective, Medicare seemed too little, too late. From the American vantage point, however, a break with tradition had apparently occurred. Some powerful constituencies had come to experience a necessity for government intervention that they had not felt before, and this necessity was recognized, in value terms, as legitimate by many others. (In the early 1960s, public opinion polls revealed that anywhere from 58% to 78% of Americans supported the idea of Medicare.)[5] How did this change come about? And why did it stop where it did? After all, if Americans over the age of 65 required federal assistance with health care costs, then it did not require an enormous leap of imagination to recognize that many people under the age of 65 required it as well. If it was incumbent on government to guarantee health care for the elderly, did it not have such a duty to the young as well? However reasonable such expectations, they were not realized—all of which frames the two critical and related questions: why did Americans come to recognize an obligation to those over 65, and why did it not culminate in national health insurance?

Many of the answers are found in the language and arguments that proponents of Medicare presented, nowhere more fully than at the extensive hearings and debates that Congress devoted to Medicare between 1963 and 1965. Surprising as it may seem, the positions adopted to establish the need for Medicare served to undermine the case for national health insurance. Proponents may have expected the measure to be the initial step on the road to such an accomplishment. But their promotion of Medicare not only failed to make the argument for national coverage but in a variety of critical ways actually subverted it. The debate made it seem as though with the exception of the elderly, no fundamental problems affected the provision of medical services in this country. Pass Medicare and seemingly all would be well in health care.

In their public presentations, the bill's advocates repeatedly distinguished Medicare from a national health insurance scheme and went to great pains to minimize the necessity for any additional interventions once the program was in place. As they offered their arguments in favor of the one measure, they simultaneously reinforced very traditional perspectives on the role of government, particularly in terms of whose interests it was to serve. Medicare was framed almost exclusively in the context of the needs and values of "the great middle class," with barely a nod to others. Perhaps the strategy represented some shrewd (if mistaken) thinking about the value of incremental gains. But Medicare proponents were themselves so focused on the needs of the middle-class elderly and so persuaded of the advantages of the marketplace for all others that they may well have believed the rhetoric that they put forward. In any event, whether it was a matter of tactics or tenet, the defense of Medicare, and the design of Medicare, made it the more likely that its passage would mark the end, not the beginning, of national health insurance.

To distinguish Medicare from national health insurance, advocates made the elderly into a special case, differentiating them from everyone else, and doing so in a manner that emphasized middle-class concerns and principles. To this end, proponents offered first an explanation of why private insurance was not adequate for those over 65, and, second, why a means test (which was a prerequisite for other welfare benefits) ought not to be required for those over 65. Third, and perhaps most challenging, they made the case for giving the elderly health care without turning it into a right that others might enjoy as well. It was a complicated assignment, for the boundary lines did not have an inherent logic of their own. The advocates managed it, but at the cost of leaving a legacy which gave only the elderly a generous and federally underwritten health care program.

From the moment the hearings opened, proponents painstakingly tried to establish that the predicament facing the elderly was special, indeed that the predicament facing the middle class elderly was special. The first statement made to the November 1963 hearings of the House Committee on Ways and Means by the secretary of health, education, and welfare, Anthony Celebrezze, laid out the grounds of the argument. Echoing the very theme that Blue Cross had used so effectively in the 1930s, Celebrezze declared that while the rich and the poor were both well served by health care services, the middle class had been ignored. "There are laws to help meet the medical expenses of those who are relatively well off through income tax deductions," he explained, "and laws that help the very poor through public assistance." But no programs assisted the middle-class majority of older people "against a real and present danger of high medical costs."[6] They had "a unique problem," confronting disproportionately higher health care costs just when their postretirement incomes were declining.

The age-specific demographic and service utilization data were easy to marshal. The elderly used health services more than others. "Nine out of ten people are hospitalized at least once after reaching age 65," Celebrezze estimated. "People over 65 use three times as much hospital care, on the average, as people under 65."[7] The elderly were twice as likely as the young to have a chronic ailment; six times as likely to be confined to their homes; seven times as likely to reside in an institution, such as a nursing home or a mental hospital. "For every 1,000 persons between the ages of 75 and 84, 83 die in a year, whereas between the ages of 25 and 34, only 1 dies of the thousand." Accordingly, "the aged spend about twice as much for physician services, over two and a half times as much for hospital care, and about 2 and a third times as much for drugs."[8]

Because the expenses associated with a hospital stay were climbing, the financial burden on the elderly was exacerbated, particularly for those who had been part of the middle class. "The costs of serious illness in old age," declared Celebrezze, "can wipe out the slender savings of a lifetime and turn security into poverty."[9] Other witnesses supplied specific dollar figures.

Hospital costs had tripled in 15 years. In 1946, the average cost of a hospital day was $9.39; in the early 1960s, it climbed to $32.28, and now was on its way to $35.[10] And surely fiscal considerations should not become the cause of depriving the elderly of in-patient care. Hospitals were no longer almshouses but temples of science, providing the latest and most advanced medical machines. "Medical technology," Celebrezze made certain to emphasize, "continues to advance and health care become not only more valuable and more important but also more expensive. It is a cruel irony that the aged, who have more than ordinary health needs and who stand to benefit the most from improvements in health care, often find this higher quality of care beyond their means."[11]

To make matters even worse for the middle-class elderly, the timing and the nature of the illnesses that affected them was altogether arbitrary. They could be healthy for years and then suddenly be struck by devastating disease. In financial terms, the greatest catastrophe, and one that apparently could not be prevented by even the most responsible and thrifty middle-class family, was a lengthy and drawn out terminal illness. As Eveline Burns of the National Consumers League explained in very class-specific terms: "This problem of the burden of medical care expenses is equally a matter of concern to people in the middle classes because of the fact that the burden is unequal. Quite frankly, sir, what we pray is that the one that is going to die first is going to die in an airplane accident or a heart attack in the economic interest of the surviving spouse."[12] It was both the strength and weakness of Medicare supporters that they personalized the issues. This was a program that they themselves needed, which made advocacy more passionate, and more value-laden.

Opponents of Medicare fought the idea of elderly exceptionalism at every turn. They tried to narrow the differences between the young and the old, not to the aim of extending Medicare coverage but of scuttling the entire program. For one, they contested generalizations about the elderly's general state of health. The spokesman for the American Medical Association, which was steadfast in its hostility, derided Medicare supporters for portraying the elderly "as universally frail and feeble, constantly ill, and doddering from one visit to the doctor to the next." In fact, they visited physicians only slightly more frequently than the young (6.8 visits a year as compared to 5).

To be sure, four out of five of the elderly had chronic conditions, but the greatest percentage of the conditions did not require confinement or cause significant limitations of activity. On average, the elderly did have longer lengths of hospital stays and incurred larger bills than those under 65. But these figures were distorted by the experience of a small minority of patients. "Ten percent of the aged," insisted the AMA testimony, "account for 39 percent of the total days of hospitalization for this age group. The same ten percent also account for about 38 percent of expenditures."[13] In other words, the scope of the problem was narrow and could be managed in targeted fashion without transforming the delivery of health care for the entire country.

Thus the debate over Medicare raised the question of whether in terms of health policy, the elderly were a distinctive group or not. The AMA had an obvious stake in saying no, insisting that small and self-contained programs could handle the marginal cases. Proponents, on the other hand, insisted that the answer was yes, in the process not only emphasizing the needs of the elderly but, and the point is crucial, minimizing the needs of everyone else. The unmistakable impression left by their testimony was that those *under* 65, regardless of class or color or age, were relatively free of the burdens caused by illness. It was only among the elderly that even the most financially prudent members of the middle class had to wish for sudden death.

The sparring that went on around age turned into open combat on the issue of middle-class access to private insurance after the age of 65. In deliberately crafted testimony, the advocates for Medicare tried to counter the proposition that the insurance system (which ostensibly worked so well for those under 65) was adequate to meet the needs of the elderly. In keeping with their overall strategy, they did not point to the general drawbacks of relying on the private sector for health insurance. They did not take note, for example, of the large numbers of low income people who were left out of the system; to make such an admission would have undercut the argument for the exceptionalism of the elderly. Instead, proponents insisted that private insurance eliminated the vulnerability of all other Americans except the elderly. The over-65 group were bereft of security because this tried and true mechanism did not work for them. Although "medical insurance has

... been urged as the answer to prayer ... for the aged middle class person," the National Consumer League testified, such purchases were often beyond their reach.[14] Or as Harrison Williams, senator from New Jersey, concluded: "Private insurance cannot do the job that must be done."[15]

In making the case against the efficacy of private insurance, Medicare's supporters argued that the price of the premiums outstripped retirement incomes. "The lowest cost private insurance programs presently available," declared New York's liberal Republican senator, Jacob Javits, "are far too expensive for most of our older citizens."[16] It required one-sixth of the median income of those over 65 to pay for coverage, thereby creating distinct financial hardships for them. The policies also typically included highly restrictive clauses, so even those who could afford to subscribe to them received less than adequate protection. Moreover, even those who had been adequately insured had to take on new policies upon retirement, and these policies often would not cover preexisting conditions. So those with a history of chronic diseases could not get protection against the very ailment whose treatment might generate exceptional expenses. To make matters even worse, these policies often set strict limits on the total dollars that would be expended or on the total number of hospital days covered. New Jersey Blue Cross, for example, provided 120 days of hospitalization for those under 65, but only 60 days to those over 65, and only 30 days for those over 70.[17] Finally, many private insurance companies wrote policies with very high deductibles, which again subscribers had to pay for from reduced retirement incomes. As a result of all these stipulations, the elderly had to pay not only expensive premiums but out-of-pocket costs of anywhere from 50% to 80% of their medical bills, and they received nothing back for nursing care.[18] "When the needs are greatest," Harrison Williams concluded, "coverage is cut." Private insurance was no alternative to Medicare.

These arguments were critical to making the case both ideologically and politically for Medicare. Were private insurance adequate to the task, there was no reason to break precedent and bring in the government to underwrite health insurance. As would therefore be expected, Medicare's opponents were desperate to refute the attack. They contended that advocates were wrong "in assuming that the middle class could not handle [the costs] and was not utilizing the private insurance technique."[19] But their counter-arguments were not very persuasive. The evidence that private insurance companies were, in fact, following restrictive strategies was simply too abundant. They, therefore, tried another tack, albeit with only modest success. Company policies, they argued, had a logic and fairness. If companies did not exclude the elderly, restrict their coverage, and charge high rates, they would be passing on the additional costs incurred to the nonelderly. They would be, as one official observed, "forcing the younger members of the community [to] pay proportionately higher premiums," thereby enabling the elderly to pay lower ones.[20] But since the issue at hand was the problems that the elderly faced, the view that the insurance policies were right in minimizing the benefits for those over 65 only served to strengthen the case for Medicare.

So intent were the champions of Medicare in demonstrating the exceptionalism of the elderly that they ignored the deficiencies of private insurance for the young. Rather than issue a broadside attack against a system of health care delivery that depended upon voluntary insurance, rather than calculate whether part-time employees could afford the rates or the deductibles, rather than analyze whether other Americans had difficulty coping with policy exclusions, Medicare's advocates made it appear as if the elderly were the only victims of these stipulations. The conclusion that Celebrezze advanced was patently untrue, but with his eye fixed on Medicare he proposed it anyway: "This combination of high health costs, low incomes, and unavailability of group insurance is what clearly distinguishes the situation of the aged as a group from the situation of younger workers as a group."[21]

Committed to this formulation, Medicare proponents persistently distorted the reality of health care delivery for those under 65. "The vast majority of young workers," declared Celebrezze, "can purchase private insurance protection." In return for bringing in government on the side of the elderly, he was ready to reject bringing it in on behalf of anyone else. "I think for younger employed people, voluntary private plans can do the job."[22]

The logic underlying these arguments was specious, although Medicare advocates never acknowledged or recognized it. It was one thing to say that those under 65 were less likely to require health care interventions; but the unasked question, of course, was, compared to whom? To say that in the aggregate the young used fewer medical services than the elderly was correct. But what about the cohort of black children, or rural residents, or low income workers? Yes, the young might be able to borrow the sums needed to meet a health emergency and pay it back after their recovery and reemployment. But that was only true for some among them, not others. It all depended on the nature of the ailment (was it time-limited with full recovery following?), access to a loan (did the person have a satisfactory career or good credit history?), and the ability to get another job, none of which could be guaranteed. Rather than confront these exceptions to their overgeneralizations, proponents simply concluded that all those below 65 could cope with health emergencies. In effect, they swept under the table the problems of access to health care for those who were temporarily or permanently outside the net of private insurance.

The second and even more difficult issue than private insurance for Medicare advocates to overcome was whether the elderly who needed assistance in health care should receive assistance through the public welfare system. After all, as one critic noted, these people had been remiss in not saving for the proverbial rainy day and the government was not obliged to intervene. Why not, in other words, hold the middle classes to their own standard? To be sure, they should not be forced to forgo health care services. But, as many opponents of Medicare, none more vigorously than the AMA, insisted, the just solution was to aid the dependent elderly through public relief. Indeed, the mechanisms were already in place to accomplish these very ends. The newly enacted Kerr-Mills program obviated the need for Medicare.

In October 1960, Congress had passed the Kerr-Mills Act, carrying the names of the powerful senator from Oklahoma, Robert Kerr, and the chairman of the House Ways and Means Committee, Wilbur Mills. The bill, as Mills later recalled, had "no opposition to it." The AMA was comfortable with this underwriting of health care so long as its provisions affected only the very poor. Medicare proponents, like Wilbur Cohen, also endorsed it on the grounds that it would accustom the public to having the federal government support health services and eventually help secure the passage of Medicare.[23]

Under the Kerr-Mills provisions, the federal government would share with the states who joined the program, the financial costs of Medical Assistance to the Aged (MAA). The details of the benefits package, including the level, type, and duration of support, were to be determined by the states; the federal government would then match from 50% to 80% of the states' expenditures. All of the participating states, however, had to set eligibility standards that required would-be enrollees (and often their adult children) to pass a means test. Recipients had to demonstrate their inability to pay medical costs by showing that their annual incomes and family assets fell below minimums fixed by the states. The standards, generally, were not as rigorous as those established for direct cash benefits under the states' welfare systems. However, the process of gaining eligibility was very much the same, requiring a formal appearance before a board and a full accounting of all resources.

As the anti-Medicare spokesmen tallied up the numbers, Kerr-Mills seemed well on its way to solving the problems of the aged who were medically indigent. By mid-1963, 28 states had joined the program, and 136,400 claimants had received $26 million in benefits. These totals, Kerr-Mills supporters noted, represented a 22% increase in claimants and a 17% increase in benefits over November 1962.[24] Thus the fact that not every state was participating in the program and that the total number of beneficiaries was still relatively low should not become a pretext for discounting its efficacy; it inevitably took time to get so complicated a state-federal alliance into place. Critics also had to remember that many of the elderly already had private insurance or other types of benefits, which obviated their need to join Kerr-Mills and reduced the number of those enrolled.[25]

The fact that Kerr-Mills benefits varied state to state, proponents contended, was no reason to condemn the program. Disparities merely reflected the fact that medical costs differed from one region to another. Moreover, there was nothing amiss in requiring a means test. "Historically," as one representative for the Chamber of Commerce told Congress, "many private and public programs providing assistance for a wide range of purposes have incorporated some form of means test to determine eligibility." The list included private and public college scholarships, student loan programs, private foundation grants, and free school lunches.[26] If these recipients had to undergo a means test, why not the aged? In short, were proponents of Medicare to show the same enthusiasm for expanding the Kerr-Mills rolls, there would be no reason to extend further government involvement in health insurance.

What made Kerr-Mills so much more attractive than Medicare to such groups as the AMA, the Chamber of Commerce, and the insurance companies was the fact that it tied benefits to poverty. In this way, private for-profit and not-for-profit companies lost no potential clients and doctors lost no paying patients, At the same time, voluntary hospitals had more of their bills paid when the indigent elderly ended up in their facilities. Thus, under Kerr-Mills, fee-for-service medicine remained alive and well and the total tax expenditures for the program were not especially heavy. Indeed, so long as government support in health care was limited to the poor, there was no ripple effect on health care policies for the larger society. Private patients were not going to clamor to enter Kerr-Mills if enrolling was tantamount to going on welfare. A government program that served the indigent would not lead to socialized medicine.[27]

The friends of Kerr-Mills were so certain of its viability that they were convinced that anyone who disagreed with them was actually intent on creating a system of national health insurance. "What we are afraid of," remarked one conservative congressman, "is the old camel's-nose-under-the-tent sort of thing. . . . Once this [Medicare] principle has been adopted . . . you will throw away the figure 65. All age limits and all medical services will be included." Now you say, "'No; we just want it over 65.' . . . Do you really think they mean it? . . . Once they get their foot in the door, that is that."[28] Were this only a question of meeting the needs of the elderly poor, the answer would rest with modest revisions to Kerr-Mills. But since the long-term agenda, opponents of Medicare believed, was national health insurance, Kerr-Mills had to be put aside and dismissed.

To counter the logic and persuasion of these arguments, Medicare supporters adopted several strategies. They not only cited the deficiencies they could identify with Kerr-Mills itself but vigorously and consistently maintained that all they truly wanted was Medicare, not national health insurance. In terms of Kerr-Mills, they insisted that it made no sense to vary health benefits state by state. Health needs transcended state boundaries, and to give more medical services to some citizens than to others was patently unfair. A resident of New York should not have better access to life-enhancing and life-preserving medical treatment than someone who lived in Mississippi. But Kerr-Mills, they noted, had been more quickly adopted in large manufacturing states than in rural ones. New York, Pennsylvania, and Illinois, not Arkansas, the Carolinas, and the Dakotas, were making it a part of their welfare programs, in this way creating obvious inequities. And some states, like Connecticut, were using the funds to reimburse convalescent and chronic disease hospitals, not to pay for acute care in general hospitals.[29] Thus, because Kerr-Mills depended on state administration, it could never meet the needs of all Americans.

To drive the larger point home and to rebut the "camel's-nose-under-the-tent" contentions, Medicare's supporters again drew rigid, and ultimately spurious, distinctions between the plight of the elderly and the predicaments that everyone else faced. Coming back to the question of holding the middle classes to their own principles, they insisted that the elderly not be forced to undergo a means test before getting health care assistance. To compel those over 65 to satisfy public welfare requirements by demonstrating their dependency was demeaning and humiliating to persons who had been independent all their adult lives. As Celebrezze exhorted: "We should do better than say to an aged person that, when he has become poor enough and when he can prove his poverty to the satisfaction of the appropriate public agency, he may be able to get help." We should take into account "the pride and independent spirit of our older people," and adopt a system which "fully safeguards the dignity and independence of our older people."[30]

The value that Celebrezze and his allies repeatedly invoked was that of dignity. "We as a nation," he declared, "owe these older people the opportunity to live their remaining years in dignity. . . . These are the types of things I am talking about, the dignity of the individual."[31] Harrison Williams, for his part, claimed that the means test provision of the Kerr-Mills program was "totally inconsistent with the dignity and sense of independence which are the right of every older American."[32] The elderly, observed Congressman Jacob Gilbert from New York, "dread the thought of having to ask for charity."[33] Or as Dr. Samuel Standard explained in countering the

AMA position: "In a country as rich as ours, shouldn't every effort be made to spare a citizen this indignity?"[34]

Many proponents believed that this sense of dignity was so critical to the middle class elderly that they would sooner forgo medical care than seek public assistance. "They are a proud lot of men and women, and they should be," declared Elmer Holland, Congressman from Pennsylvania. "Rather than do what is required, such as bring their children into court, have a lien placed on their home, display their financial need for medical care at the office of the department of public assistance, these men and women will go without necessary care."[35] Fully 12 of the 28 states participating in Kerr-Mills, added Gilbert, required that the relatives of the elderly undergo a means test before assistance was allowed, and he, too, was convinced that the elderly would forgo needed medical care before they would bring their children into the welfare system, or force their children to pay their medical bills.[36]

The labor unions that lined up in support of Medicare (which had no negative consequences for their influence, since benefits affected retirees) were particularly active in combating the notion that indigency should be required before assistance was granted. As a representative of the International Ladies Garment Workers Union told Congress: "The rise of a new phrase, 'medical indigency,' does not remove the stigma of charity from this program."[37] Thus Kerr-Mills would never serve the majority of the elderly, and union programs and funds would have to continue to carry a burden that was becoming more onerous. "Our costs have mounted," complained one American Federation of Labor spokesman, "far beyond our most pessimistic expectations. . . . We are convinced by our own experience that no single, isolated group of American workers can, on its own, provide indefinitely for the extraordinary costs of decent health care for its retired citizens."[38] Left to Kerr-Mills, the middle-class elderly would suffer, and so would the middle-class employees whose wages would be reduced in order to pay for their own health insurance and that of the retirees as well.

These points were well taken and, in many instances, accurate. But if the process of obtaining welfare was so humiliating an experience, why should *anyone* have to suffer the procedure? If it constituted so fundamental an affront to the dignity of the elderly, why was it not also an affront to the dignity of the young? To which the tacit answer was the well-worn one that as a rule, the poor had only themselves to blame. The elderly apart, welfare recipients were "unworthy," which implied that humiliation was their due, at least until they reached the age of 65.[39]

Thus the positions adopted to promote Medicare reinforced the most traditional and negative attitudes about poverty and welfare. To be sure, advocates could not fight every battle at once and on all fronts, and they were forced into this line of argument by the need to rebut claims that Kerr-Mills could substitute effectively for Medicare. But they succumbed all too easily, sharing more of the conventional ideology than they were ready to admit. Rather than try to generalize the discourse, to note that welfare might also be an affront to anyone waiting for hours on a relief line and suffering the hostile looks and aggressive questions of a suspicious case worker, they urged that the elderly, but only the elderly, be exempted from the process. Everyone else on welfare apparently received the scrutiny they deserved.

Finally, by limiting their advocacy to the elderly and not to all Americans, Medicare proponents had to hedge the question of whether health care was a right due all citizens. It was very tempting to rest a federal health insurance program for the elderly on the premise that "the Federal Government, as a matter of right, owes medical care to elderly people." On these grounds, the means test stipulations of Kerr-Mills were obviously improper; in fact, the entire case for Medicare became the simpler to formulate and defend. Over the course of their congressional testimony, advocates did occasionally slip into the language of rights. Celebrezze opened his testimony with the declaration: "What is required as the first line of defense, is protection furnished as a right."[40] So, too, New York's mayor, Robert Wagner, shared with his liberal constituents a belief that "medical care in their old age . . . is a matter of right."

But to assert that health care was truly a right meant that restricting benefits to those over 65 was improper, or that the new legislation, just as opponents had feared, was a way station to a more inclusive program. The typical route out of the dilemma was for Medicare advocates to rebut the proposition that health care was a right, to deny that the federal government owed anyone "medical attention as a right." Instead, they adopted the position that Medicare benefits would be paid for by the recipients during their working years, and to this end, they made Medicare part of the Social Security system, not a program standing alone.

Linking Medicare to Social Security had a number of advantages which proponents found irresistible, and some disadvantages that they were prepared to live with. For one, by the mid-1960s, Social Security had lost the controversial character that it had when Franklin Roosevelt first proposed it. Public opinion polls reported overwhelming public satisfaction with the program; no one thought that the sums paid out to recipients had anything to do with federal social welfare assistance or for that matter, with big government itself. Thus, making Medicare part of Social Security enabled Congressmen like Jacob Gilbert to describe the new legislation as providing an "earned right." His colleague from Wisconsin initially claimed that medical care for the aged should be provided to "our citizens as a right, not as a privilege"; but he immediately qualified, really contradicted, this proposition by adding that since the benefits would come through Social Security, "individual citizens earn their right to a decent retirement by virtue of their contributions during their working years."[41]

An "earned right" was an odd formulation, to say the least, confounding contract obligations with essential principles. But it did link Medicare to one of the most popular federal programs. Opponents came back with a mere quibble: while 20 years hence it might be true that recipients had paid for their medical insurance through Social Security, the first beneficiaries had surely not. To which Medicare champions responded that even if the first recipients would not have paid for their benefits in strict actuarial terms, still they had made their contributions "on a total program basis."[42] Although the meaning of that phrase was altogether obscure, the force of the argument was not: Americans could enjoy Medicare without buying into national health insurance. The principle remained that one received what one paid for, more or less.

Linking Medicare to Social Security reinforced in still other ways the contention that the change was self-contained, and not the opening thrust in a larger campaign. Because Medicare was to be entirely self-financing, paid for from employee contributions and administered through a specially created trust fund, there would be no incentive, or capacity, to extend coverage to the unemployed, or to lower the age of eligibility. By the same token, and despite their derisive comments about Kerr-Mills, Medicare supporters assured the opposition that they intended to keep that program in place. The elderly who needed services not covered by Medicare would have to turn to Kerr-Mills for relief.[43] The trade-off, again, had the least negative impact on the middle classes. In effect, reformers, by their own terms, were advancing the needs of the middle-class elderly by sacrificing the dignity of the lower-class elderly. For those with the least resources, a means test and a forced declaration of pauperism in order to obtain health services apparently was not demeaning.

Making other attempts to persuade opponents that Medicare was not a forerunner of national health insurance, supporters accepted still more compromises in the administration of the program—compromises that, again, were not injurious to the middle classes. Thus, proponents did not object to levying deductibles before benefits began; these initial charges would not be nearly as onerous to the middle-class elderly as to those living on more reduced postretirement incomes. By the same token, Medicare's coverage was initially limited to hospital bills and excluded physicians' services. Here, too, the financial impact on the middle-class elderly was substantially less than on the lower-class elderly.

In still other ways, Medicare's advocates countered, all too effectively as it turned out, charges of incrementalism. The day-to-day management of Medicare was given over to the voluntary sector, namely, Blue Cross, a tactic designed both to placate opponents of "big government," and to assure organized medicine that Medicare would not bring with it governmental regulation and oversight of medical practices. Moreover, Medicare agreed to pay physicians' fees on the basis of "customary and reasonable" charges— the most generous possible formulation. (Not surprisingly, physician incomes skyrocketed after Medicare, and for the first time, medicine become a lucrative profession.)

Finally, almost by coincidence but with profound implications for the future role of government in health care, the passage of Medicare became the occasion to pass Medicaid. The two programs could not have been more different, and these very differences helped to ensure that the principles of Medicare would not be applied more broadly.

Medicaid, as the scholars of the field know well but others often forget, was a legislative afterthought, inserted by Wilbur Mills into the legislative package with little debate or public discussion. Its provisions resembled those of Kerr-Mills, applied now to all of the poor, not just the elderly. Eligibility criteria (beyond the fact that recipients had to pass a means test) and the extent of the benefits and services provided were left to the states to determine, with the federal government matching the state appropriations. Medicaid was, in every sense, a traditional welfare measure, distrustful of the poor and more concerned with screening out miscreants than delivering services. Its linkage to Medicare testified not to a generosity of spirit or heightened recognition of the fundamental values of health care but to yet another round in the battle to restrict the principles of Medicare to those over 65. This is precisely why Medicaid was endorsed by the AMA and put forward by Mills himself. It was an insurance policy to make certain that the next generation of reformers could not marshall the arguments in favor of Medicare and contend that they were equally applicable to those below 65![44]

Clearly, all these maneuvers were part of a strategy to get Medicare enacted, whatever the eventual price to a national health insurance program. So long as the system of private insurance purchased through the marketplace remained at the core of health policy and the special needs of the middle classes were met, the results were favorable. Medicare proponents took the pragmatic route, unwilling to endorse a right to health care, afraid to advocate for a program in terms that were more universal than middle-class interests.

In the end, it was the 1930s almshouse dynamic revisited. Because the worthy middle class could not be expected to go on relief to gain medical benefits, the system had to bend, but only part way. Medicare would protect the elderly middle classes from burdensome costs, not break new ground in conceptualizing health care rights. Thus, the elderly became, and remained (with the one exception that we will turn to next) the only group with federally guaranteed access to health care.

4 Dialysis and National Priorities

The history of kidney dialysis starkly exemplifies the increasing strains between the two fundamental tenets of the American credo in health care: unfettered middle-class access to technology in a system that relies essentially on the marketplace to provide health care coverage. Medicare made manifest one fissure: the private sector was not capable of meeting the overall needs of the elderly. The dialysis experience exposed a second. Like the iron lung, the dialysis machine was able to compensate for the failure of a vital organ, enabling patients with end-stage renal disease to survive. But the technology was so expensive and scarce as to stand beyond the reach of the middle classes and their philanthropic organizations. To ameliorate this desperate situation, in effect to satisfy what was perceived to be middle-class needs, the federal government intervened. In 1972, Congress agreed to underwrite all the costs of treating end-stage kidney disease and to this day kidney failure is the only ailment with its own guaranteed funding stream.

The glaring inconsistency in policy—why single out end-stage kidney disease for preferential treatment?—was even more difficult to justify than the passage of Medicare. The elderly, at least, were a more broadly based group than those suffering from kidney disease. Proponents tried a variety of strategies, including one that defended the special program as a step toward national health insurance. But again the expectation proved fanciful, and the dialysis precedent, like Medicare, turned into a negative reference point for health policy. For the first time, a number of critics began to tally up the costs, economic and social, of the ardent American romance with medical machines. Their calculations suggested that government could not satisfy demands in health care. Americans were going to have to change their attitudes and practices in fundamental ways.

Just as physicians before the invention of the iron lung had been able to respond to short-term but not chronic episodes of respiratory failure, so, too, before kidney dialysis, they had been able to treat acute but not permanent loss of kidney functioning. During World War II, William Kolff, working in the Netherlands under German occupation, devised a method and a machine to filter a patient's blood through a cellophane tubing and clean it of impurities. He began using the procedure in 1943; the first 16 of his patients died, but the 17th lived, his body cleansed of uremia. After the war, Kolff built several of his machines and sent them abroad. He also came to the United States and worked with engineers and physicians at Boston's Peter Brent Brigham hospital to build what became known as the Kolff-Brigham machine. From 1947 to 1960, physicians used it to treat acute and temporary injury to the kidney. But there was little they could do for the patient with chronic kidney failure because each time a patient required the intervention, a surgeon had to cut into an artery and a vein so as to divert the flow of blood through the cellophane filter and then back into the body. Within a matter of weeks, the surgeon would have exhausted the available blood vessel sites and could do nothing more. Thus the Kolff technique was able to tide a patient over until the organ recovered. But if the organ was permanently damaged, the treatment was useless.[1]

In 1960, Dr. Belding Scribner of the University of Washington Medical School transformed dialysis from a short-term to a long-term treatment. He designed a permanent in-dwelling cannula and shunt that permitted a patient to be easily connected and reconnected to the dialysis machine, plugged in as it were, without the need for additional surgery. The critical material in his machine was Teflon, discovered accidentally in 1938 at a Du Pont laboratory. Teflon was so inert chemically that the body did not reject it and thereby tolerated the in-dwelling cannula. (Its inert quality soon made it highly attractive to consumers in the form of Teflon-coated frying pans.) Thus, over the course of an eight-hour dialysis session, the patient's blood circulated through the machine and, with the assistance of the Teflon, was cleansed of the impurities. Patients with chronic end-stage renal disease (ESRD) could undergo this treatment two or three times a week and thereby remain alive and functioning for many years.

The dialysis machine, like the iron lung, was born of clinical necessity. Before his innovation, Scribner could use a Kolff-like intervention to save a patient from imminent death but was unable to treat those with irreversible organ failure. As he recalls, he brought one acutely ill patient back to life, did a biopsy on his kidneys, and learned that they were both destroyed. "So we had to go through the trauma of telling his wife that despite the amazing recovery she still must take him home to die a second time." Deeply disturbed by these events, Scribner found himself returning again and again to the problem, searching for a permanent solution. A few weeks later, "I literally woke up in the middle of the night with the idea of how we could save these people."[2]

Scribner's breakthrough did not immediately improve the life chances of many patients with ESRD. In 1969, only some 1000 patients were receiving dialysis. By 1973, right before the new federal reimbursement policy became effective, the number had increased to approximately 10,000; ten years later it would stand at 65,000.[3] Part of the reason for the lag in dialysis treatment was the cost of opening, staffing, and equipping a new center; part of it, too, was that physicians were not trained to the techniques and, to a degree, were not eager to learn. (They much preferred to cure acute cases than attend to chronic ones.) In all events, for over a decade patients with end-stage kidney disease outnumbered the machines and centers available to treat them.

The first team to cope with the issue of distributing a scarce, life-saving resource was Scribner's. To resolve the dilemma of who would receive life-saving access to dialysis, it asked the Seattle medical society to appoint a lay committee of seven "quite ordinary people" to determine "life or death." The team would first screen all candidates and identify those who were medically and psychiatrically appropriate for the procedure. But because there were many more potential beneficiaries than machines, the lay committee would have to make the final choice.[4]

The lay committee first decided to restrict beneficiaries to residents of Washington State—on the dubious ethical and factual grounds that since the state's tax dollars had supported the research, only its citizens should reap the rewards. But that still left four candidates for every one dialysis place. To narrow the list further, the committee proceeded on frankly utilitarian grounds. It would provide access to the machine to those most likely to benefit the community, and it went on to define "benefits" in highly conventional terms. It gave preference to the employed over the unemployed, to a parent over a nonparent, to the married over the single, to churchgoers over atheists, and to law-abiding citizens over the deviant. Speaking in June 1963, Scribner reported that over the last year, "The lay committee accepted ten and rejected seven. All the latter group died."[5]

The dilemma that Seattle faced soon spread as other institutions obtained their own dialysis equipment. To cope with demands, New York's Downstate Medical Center emulated Seattle by establishing a lay committee to judge potential patients in terms of their social worth. Other medical centers adopted a principle of first come, first served, or tried to reserve treatment for those most desperately ill. But whatever the formula adopted, no one was satisfied with the process or the results. These were hard choices that made everyone uncomfortable.[6]

American medicine might possibly have continued to muddle through the problem of allocating the scarce dialysis resource without provoking hostile reactions. Perhaps, with time, the pressures from patients would abate as more machines and medical centers became capable of treating kidney failure. And, in truth, dialysis did have drawbacks. As with the iron lung, physicians, and some patients too, expressed misgivings about the desirability and efficacy of the treatment. For one, the intervention was very expensive. Excluding capital expenditures to make space available for the equipment, the annual cost of dialysis in the 1970s, per hospital patient, was approximately $20,000.

Dialysis was (and is) a form of chronic care, which typically has a low priority in the American medical system. Dialysis, like the iron lung, earned the frankly disparaging epithet, from Lewis Thomas, of a "half-way technology." Since it did not cure the disease or add to knowledge about its etiology, it merely represented a means of coping. For this very reason, Thomas, and others as well, urged that dialysis not be permitted to deplete medical resources, and, consistent with this advice, a number of tertiary care institutions, including Columbia-Presbyterian Medical Center, refrained from opening dialysis units. Far better to search for cures than invest heavily in chronic care.

Even more telling, dialysis brought with it serious side effects, both physiological and psychological. As described in medical journals (but not so often, as we shall see, in the popular press), dialysis required that patients restrict their diets. They had to exclude all salt and minimize protein intake — meat was almost forbidden; they could drink only one glass of water a day and no alcohol at all. Between dialysis sessions, patients frequently suffered from headaches and general fatigue; some even experienced excruciating itching. All the while, they had to spend some 30 hours a week on the machine, a process that left them physically drained. According to one survey, almost half of patients undergoing dialysis were too enervated to hold a job.

The machines also rendered some patients psychologically dependent on the technology itself, on the technicians that ran them, or, in the case of home dialysis, on family members. This dependence exacted its own price in the form of depression and divorce; surveys reported that as many as one-third of dialysis patients had contemplated suicide. The treatment itself was not free of medical complications. Depending on the age and general health of the patient, mortality rates on dialysis fluctuated between 5% and 20% annually. Death could come from bleeding, hepatitis, hypertension, pulmonary embolus, or infection.[7]

As would be expected, the dialysis machine, again in the tradition of the iron lung, generated its full share of nightmarish images. If the iron lung was coffinlike, the dialysis machine was more simply, "the monster." Although not all patients carried such dark images of themselves and the machine, some felt the burden of treatment very deeply. One wrote about being tethered to the machine as though they were partners in an unholy marriage: "The Travenol [dialysis machine] salesman wearing glasses and a dark suit: 'Do you take this machine in sickness and in health till death do you part?' I do." Another protested:

> I am the final essence of the technological age,
> Flesh conjoined with plastic, vessels with steel,
> Coils, alarms, twisted tubing turning scarlet.
> Deep within the machine dark blood
> Mixing with fluid, cellophane separated, plugged in and turned on.
> Dear God Purify me.[8]

In psychiatric interviews, some patients referred to themselves as the "living dead," and bluntly described their abhorrence of the machine. As one case record read: "She expressed considerable hatred of the machine, endowing it with human motives. She referred to it vehemently . . . as 'that hateful thing.' . . . I sometimes feel like destroying it.'" Another patient conceded that without the machine she "wouldn't be here to write this and yet I find it impossible to make friends with the monster." And still other patients thought of themselves as Frankenstein's offspring, their shunts giving them the appearance of his monster.[9]

Were all these desperate and despairing reactions not sufficient to stifle enthusiasm for dialysis and make the question of adequate supply seem less pressing, Americans could look abroad and find persuasive evidence of the feasibility and seeming ethical propriety of restricting access to the machine. Although dialysis technology spread quickly to England and the European continent, physicians in most of these countries were highly selective in their choice of patients; indeed, they continued to be selective even as the number of machines proliferated. British physicians were particularly parsimonious. They would not refer older patients or patients suffering from other serious diseases for dialysis treatment. They would not even inform many patients about this option to prolong their lives.

In all, there were many compelling objections to making a massive commitment to dialysis, including cost, chronicity, and poor quality of life. In policy terms, the technology could have been treated as one that merely prolonged the process of dying—a position, which, in fact had strong advocates. Peter Salisbury, the founder of the American Society for Artificial Organs, concluded (perhaps reflecting his own professional interests) that dialysis represented little more than the "palliative treatment of incurable diseases." Others insisted that: "Dying would be a lesser evil than the treatment proposed." It would not have been unthinkable for American physicians to emulate their British counterparts in limiting access to dialysis.

But this was not the course followed. Rather than adopt strategies to ration dialysis, American social policy set out to ensure that the technology was available to everyone who needed it. Under Section 2991 of the Social Security Act of 1972, the treatment of end-stage renal disease became the first (and only) disease for which the U. S. Congress agreed to underwrite all costs of care. Instead of formulating restrictions on the use of the technology, social policy guaranteed open access. The decision raises in stark fashion the question of why Americans insisted on making the dialysis machine readily available. Why did access to this technology, like the iron lung before it, have to be democratized?

The answer begins with an appreciation of how "technology creep" works in American society. Even before the advent of federal funding, in 1973, the number of dialysis machines and dialysis centers had increased, although supply continued to fall short of demand. By 1969, as as noted above, approximately 1000 patients were receiving dialysis in the United States, and these 1000 patients represented a constituency that would work both to obtain reimbursement for their expenses and, with only slightly less enthusiasm, to encourage an expansion of the number of dialysis centers. "Before 1973," as a report of the Institute of Medicine on dialysis policy makes clear, "patients were disproportionately white, middle-class men with high educational status," in effect, those best situated and most likely to agitate successfully for a new policy.[10] And joining patients in this drive were physicians, particularly specialists in nephrology, hospital administrators, nurses, and families and friends of the patients themselves. In short order, dialysis created a cadre of laymen and professionals who had a profound stake in the machine.

The very existence of both this technology and constituency encouraged, at times even compelled, still others to support its spread. Consider, for example, the predicament confronting Dr. Harold Schnaper, of the U. S. Veterans Administration. In 1963, at a medical conference on dialysis, Schnaper announced that the VA had received a request from a number of its physicians that it establish a chronic dialysis unit in Los Angeles. Recognizing that "this was the first of a large number of requests," Schnaper explained that VA hospitals were beginning to open dialysis centers around the country. "How far the VA will be able to go in the dialysis contract still requires scrutiny," he commented "but I do want the audience to know that within the next three years, the VA will have 30 centers in operation."[11]

Why did the VA decide to provide the units when dialysis was still more of an experimental procedure than proven therapy? Because VA administrators were not going to allow themselves to be questioned, or criticized, for denying the veterans of America's wars access to a life-saving technology. If the question was "who lives and who dies?" the answer could not be that those who die are those who fought for their country. Confronting scarcity, the VA defined its role as making certain that its own constituency did not lose out. Moreover, the VA decision was not an excruciating one to reach, at least in terms of direct financial considerations. Relatively well funded by Congress, the VA did not have to decide what alternative programs might have to be reduced or eliminated in order to include dialysis.

The VA's very ability to treat dialysis as an add-on and not worry about trade-offs was fully appreciated by officials outside its administration, and obviously worried them. The Bureau of the Budget, the arm of the federal government charged to think about cost containment and triage among scarce resources, was particularly upset. In order to formulate a response, the bureau convened a committee to examine the need for dialysis programs; anticipating that the consensus would be against the policy, it would then have the ammunition to recommend against an enlarged VA program.

To the bureau's acute disappointment, the report enthusiastically endorsed the technology and encouraged greater investments in it.[12] The committee, chaired by Carl Gottschalk, a nephrologist and professor of medicine at the University of North Carolina, and composed predominantly of physicians, first resolved that dialysis worked well—it was no longer experimental. Despite some severe side effects, it constituted a highly effective therapy. The committee then went on to urge a major commitment to kidney dialysis. The technology is "sufficiently well advanced today to warrant launching a national program intended to provide such treatment for those medically suitable patients."[13] As befit the ethics of the medical profession and as might be expected from a group that had no direct stake or concern for federal budget deficits, the committee espoused the principle that if the lives of some patients could be saved, then the investment had to be made. It calculated that some 8000 patients required dialysis but only 1750 were now receiving it. In human terms, this meant that some 6000 Americans a year were dying needlessly. Thus the step from the VA adding dialysis to its services to a national commission urging still more investment in dialysis was quickly made. The Bureau of the Budget, for the obvious reasons, tried to bury the report—one wonders why it ever thought a medical committee would decide otherwise—but it could not contain the policy recommendations expressed.

At the same time, patient groups grew stronger and more aggressive because of the life-and-death stakes involved and because the procedures for delivering dialysis were ideally suited to foster group consciousness and advocacy among middle-class men. They all received initial treatment in hospital units or large centers. These units, equipped with anywhere from 4 to 12 machines, dialyzed patients simultaneously, in a process that took six to eight hours and occurred regularly three times a week. The regimen thus guaranteed that patients would get to know each other intimately, and have ample occasion to discuss the full range of problems, including financial ones, that they all faced.

Just how tailor-made the situation was for stimulating patient advocacy is apparent in the formation of the National Association of Patients on Hemodialysis (NAPH), a group that played a critical role in the passage of Section 2991 of the 1972 Social Security Act. NAPH, the counterpoint in kidney disease to the National Foundation for Infantile Paralysis in polio, was the brainstorm of four patients who dialyzed together at Kings County Hospital in Brooklyn, New York. In fact, over the first several years of its existence, the group used Kings County for its mailing address. At its moment of founding, the NAPH president, Samuel Orenstein, a lawyer, had been on dialysis for six years. The vice president and the editor of its newsletter, William Blackton, a Columbia College graduate and aspiring journalist, had been on dialysis for four years. The two treasurers of the organization had each been dialyzed at Kings County for five years. William Cohen, who served as legal counselor and lobbyist for the group, was the exception—he underwent dialysis at home.

As befit a patient group, NAPH opened its membership only to those on dialysis. And as befit the middle-class and professional credentials of its organizers, one of NAPH's first activities was to publish a newsletter that reported the latest developments in dialysis technology, from changes in the design of shunts to anticlotting drugs. It also included advice on strategies and opportunities for vacation travel. Since patients could not be more than two or three days away from dialysis equipment, the newsletter supplied information on how to arrange for dialysis in Hawaii (one year's notice was required), or in France (staffs there were particularly efficient), or anywhere else (by contacting fellow dialysis patients and arranging to use their equipment). The letters to the editor section, like those that appeared in patient newspapers in chronic diseases hospitals, particularly tuberculosis sanatoriums, mixed accounts of good cheer with shared pain. The NAPH also published recipes for salt-free cookies and recounted with pride how one dialysis patient made it through the rigors of medical school and internship.

However useful these columns were to middle-class subscribers (who else was interested in how to dialyze in France?), the NAPH was not mainly concerned in spreading information. The primary focus of the newsletter, and at the core of the organization's activities, was political action. Its goal was not to raise charitable contributions to offset the cost of dialysis—the NAPH model was not the March of Dimes. Perhaps it was because of the precedent of Medicare—a government that intervened for the elderly should intervene for the kidney patient—or because of the size of the required expenditures—dialysis machines and treatment were far more costly than iron lungs. Whatever the reason, the NAPH had recourse to Washington, not to local communities and philanthropists. Thus the first issue of its newsletter pledged that the "NAPH will represent the interests of dialysis patients in local, state and federal governments," particularly in supporting bills to obtain funding to cover all the costs of dialysis. And to make its case, the first flier that the founders mailed to some 200 dialysis centers opened with the lines, taken directly from the Gottschalk report: "100,000 people die from kidney disease each year in the U. S. 10,000 of these people could be saved if they could get artificial kidney treatments. But there just aren't enough machines available. So, thousands die *needlessly* each year because of a simple lack of equipment."

As befit a middle-class group aiming its arguments at mainstream America, the NAPH adopted a position, repeated again and again in its newsletter and in its Congressional testimony, that dialysis posed no problems for the rich—they could purchase their own home equipment—or for the poor—who could often obtain reimbursement for dialysis from public welfare programs. Just like the earlier proponents of Blue Cross and Medicare, the NAPH spokesmen argued that only the middle classes were disadvantaged. They had too many personal resources to qualify for welfare but not enough to cover the cost of dialysis. They could not themselves meet the $20,000 cost of dialysis in hospitals or the expenses for home dialysis (with a price of $15,000 to $20,000 for a machine and annual maintenance costs of some $5000 to $6000).[14] Even those fortunate enough to have private insurance learned that many companies, including Blue Cross in New York, did not reimburse for home dialysis.

Accordingly, the NAPH favored any and all initiatives that would provide reimbursement for dialysis. It informed its membership about pending health care legislation, identified the chairpersons of the relevant House and Senate committees, and urged letter writing campaigns. The advice to patients and families to lobby and to write was well received. On one item of legislation NAPH members did everything from gathering signatures at suburban shopping centers to getting the Pearl Harbor Survivors Club to write supporting letters. As a result, one Congressman reported that he had received 10,000 letters the previous week on the bill, and 90% of them were favorable.[15]

The NAPH leadership also garnered support from notable citizens who had a special interest in kidney disease, usually because of the illness of a close relative or friend. In this way, Mrs. Ralph Bunche came to serve as honorary chairman of the NAPH—her husband had been on dialysis for six months before his death in December 1971.

To these same ends, the NAPH consistently championed national health insurance bills. From its moment of inception, it linked the particular needs of dialysis patients to a still wider cause. That so middle class an organization actively promoted national health insurance should not be surprising. It reflects the unusual circumstance that its members confronted: illness, if you will, trumps class considerations. Unlike most others in the middle class, dialysis patients were not protected by private insurance from potentially devastating medical costs; and by virtue of the fact that they were all under 65, they were not eligible for Medicare benefits.[16] Thus their advocacy is the exception that proves the rule. Absent a critical need such as dialysis, the middle classes had no personal stake in federal intervention. Or to put this conclusion in terms of the general maxim that we have been exploring: when private insurance is insufficient to meet middle-class medical needs, particularly when access to advanced technology is at stake, then, but only then, will middle-class advocacy for government intervention flourish.

Recognizing that the prospects for national health insurance were dim, the NAPH ultimately devoted the bulk of its energies to promoting the specific needs of dialysis patients. It fought with insurance companies, like New York's Blue Cross, to have them alter reimbursement policies and cover home dialysis. It even threatened to picket Blue Cross offices if it did not change its policies. The NAPH also held press conferences to make the case that home dialysis was much cheaper than hospital-based dialysis, rebutting arguments that such a benefit would increase insurance costs. The tactics worked. Early in 1972, New York's Blue Cross agreed to cover home dialysis.[17]

The NAPH was only one of the many organizations that lobbied on behalf of kidney patients. The National Kidney Association, under the leadership of Dr. George Schreiner of the Georgetown University Medical School, was an especially active advocate in Washington. The Kidney Association, however, unlike the NAPH, was physician-dominated and, therefore, interested not only in promoting patient care but in securing appropriations for research into kidney disease. There were also dozens of smaller patient groups, including People on Artificial Kidneys (in New Jersey, Delaware, and Pennsylvania), and the Kidney Foundation (in Illinois), promoting their concerns before state legislatures as well as Congress.[18]

The overall impact of all these efforts is not easy to measure, but the groups certainly won a substantial number of victories. On the local level and step-by-step, they were establishing the legislative basis for a more comprehensive program. By 1970, 21 states had made appropriations of over $5 million annually for kidney disease; New York, Illinois, and Pennsylvania were in the lead.[19] To be sure, fund-raising drives (from bake sales to raffles) never matched the professionalism and success of the March of Dimes. But the kidney organizations were able to raise public sympathy for the plight of dialysis patients.

No matter how energetic and effective the lobbying conducted by patient advocates and impressive the incremental gains that they achieved in legislatures, they were not in themselves sufficient to persuade the federal government to single out end-stage renal disease and provide all the costs of its care. Many other worthy ventures, within and without medicine, clamored for support; self-interested patient groups, even when they attract powerful allies, can take legislative proposals just so far. Rather, to understand the victories that kidney patients won, it is vital to reckon with their ability to devise a broader, societywide appeal. It was not the strength of their particular lobbying efforts but their ability to tie their own cause into the American credo in health care that brought them victories. In effect, the campaign for democratizing access to the machine was successful because it was able to appeal to basic values within the American system.

From Dr. Scribner's innovation in 1960 to the passage of Section 2991 of the Social Security Act of 1972, the problem of allocating dialysis machines to all who needed them captured exceptional public attention. In editorial pages, television programs, scholarly journals, academic conferences, congressional hearings, and congressional debates, a powerful consensus emerged that considered the prospect of rationing this life-preserving medical technology to be intolerable.[20]

This conclusion reflected, first, a fundamental hostility to the idea of using ad hoc committees to make life–death decisions. The Seattle procedures captured notoriety in Shana Alexander's widely-read 1962 *Life* magazine article, "They Decide Who Lives." Having attended the committee meetings, Alexander reported with little editorial comment on how members unabashedly invoked social criteria to reach their judgments, readily advancing the candidacy of patients who were most like them (that is, married, hard-working, public service oriented, and family-minded), and denying access to the machine to the others. Soon, commentators, coming from the growing ranks of philosophers and lawyers who were becoming interested in medical decision making, addressed the dubious ethicality of such criteria. (Indeed, some historians date the origins of the bioethics movement to this episode.) Thus the authors of one Law Review article found the account of the Seattle deliberations "numbing." They went on to ask: "What is meant by 'public service'? Were the people who got themselves jailed in the South while working for civil rights doing a 'public service'? What about working for the Antivivisection League?" In what was the single best line to emerge from the debate, they aptly concluded: "The Pacific Northwest is no place for a Henry David Thoreau with bad kidneys."[21]

Physicians also voiced their objections to so-called who-shall-live committees. "Many newsmen and television writers have relished dramatizing the decision," complained one New York nephrologist in the *Journal of the*

American Medical Association. "But what they don't realize is that . . . there is nothing heroic, ennobling, or even dramatic about such a situation; if anything it is degrading and pathetic."[22] Or as consultants to the National Kidney Foundation concluded: "It is neither morally nor politically acceptable, and perhaps not legally permissible, to allow one class of persons to live and another to die. Yet, that is precisely what is happening."[23]

Elected officials echoed these same opinions. Vance Hartke, senator from Indiana and one of the key sponsors of legislation on behalf of dialysis patients, considered who-shall-live committees nothing less than "intolerable."[24] Immediately before the vote on the 1972 legislation, he had inserted into the *Congressional Record* a fact sheet on dialysis and a *New York Times* article both of which were highly critical of the Seattle proceedings. Henry Jackson, senator from Washington State, also expressed his displeasure: "I think it is a great tragedy, in a nation as affluent as ours, that we have to consciously make a decision all over America as to the people who will live and the people who will die. We had a committee in Seattle . . . who had to pass judgment on who would live and who would die. I believe we can do better than that."[25]

An emphasis on the particular characteristics of dialysis patients encouraged this perspective. In the congressional hearings and debates, the patients were consistently identified as young and productive citizens who would be able to lead fully normal lives if they had access to the technology. The characterization was demographically correct; in the early 1970s, but not, as we shall see, two decades later, patients on dialysis were almost all between the ages of 15 and 55.[26] But what is most notable is the way that this fact was framed. Senator Hartke, for example, insisted that "sixty percent of those on dialysis can return to work but require retraining and most of the remaining 40 percent need no retraining whatsoever."[27] And dialysis, everyone agreed, worked well; the procedure had long ago lost its experimental status. Hence, those who died from ESRD were "elective deaths," that is, patients who had been "allowed to die," or "permitted to die."[28] Or, in the most dramatic of the phrases, these were people who "die needlessly."[29]

Advocates for the dialysis patients also had little difficulty in presenting the "who-shall-live" committees, in general, and the shortage of a lifesaving technology, in particular, not only as scandalous but unprecedented.

After all, the iron lung had been widely available, and other interventions, including drugs like penicillin, had been rationed only for a brief period of time. Dr. Samuel Kountz, professor of medicine from the University of California, San Francisco, and a leader of the National Kidney Disease Foundation, testified before Congress that dialysis represented a "national crisis in medicine unparalleled in our history. . . . Today, physicians are forced to stand silently by and let their patients die when they know a proven form of treatment exists, which if it could be made available would save their lives." Concluded Kountz: "Never before has a proven lifesaving treatment been denied to so many primarily because of the lack of money." In all, thousands of people a year were "dying needlessly."[30]

As public debate over dialysis intensified, it became increasingly difficult to accept the idea that money was sufficient reason to allow a group defined as young and productive to die. The very idea that this could happen in the United States inevitably provoked angry commentaries about wasteful spending. The dialysis story served as a tablet on which could be inscribed one's favorite frivolous expenditure. Thus Senator Hartke found it unconscionable that in a country so saturated with consumer goods, a life-saving machine might remain in short supply; a society dedicated to consumption could not stop at the hospital door. "Tens of billions of dollars," declared Hartke, "are spent on . . . cosmetics to make us look pleasing, and on appliances to make our lives easier. . . . We can begin to set our national priorities by a national effort to bring kidney disease treatment within the reach of all those in need." The concept of America as bountiful could not be so blatantly contradicted.

Once the line was sharply drawn between money and life, the answer in a democratically elected political forum had to be life. No politician would wish to defend the proposition that the rich could live because they had access to a machine, while the middle class died because they could not afford it. One might ask why a similar reaction did not promote preventive health measures, or to move down the social scale, why when comparative statistics demonstrated unequivocally that the rich lived longer than the poor and that rates of mortality in black ghettos were many times greater than those in other communities, no reforms were initiated, including national health insurance? The answers, however, are relatively clear. For one, the middle-class character of the dialysis advocates and dialysis patients was a distinct advantage. For another, statistical overviews can never match the power of the particular case. Here one was not presenting averages or epidemiological trends, but advocating for specific people.

Indeed, proponents made certain to present the predicament of those suffering from ESRD in terms of named individuals, almost always drawn from the middle classes. Note, for example, the life histories of those who appeared before a House committee in 1971 to buttress the point that access to dialysis meant life or death: for William Litchfield ("You can see by the very presence of us today that . . . persons [on dialysis] . . . can lead a relatively normal life"); for Mrs. June Crowley (mother of four, one of whom wants to become a doctor, another, a marine biologist); and for Abraham Holtz (working full-time as an accountant, with only occasional time off for a check-up).[31] This was not just a statistical cohort at risk, but people like you and me.

To the same end of personalizing and dramatizing the issue, Shep Glaser actually underwent dialysis in the congressional committee room. Glaser, vice president and later president of the NAPH, had the cooperation of a kidney specialist at nearby Georgetown; and although his appearance was delayed because of a sudden drop in his blood pressure, he entered the committee room hooked up to a dialysis machine and explained how the procedure worked. While some might consider this an unfortunate publicity stunt, it had an extraordinarily favorable effect. One House member called it a "very impressive demonstration . . . on something that there has been a lot of misconception about." Another confessed: "I don't know of any testimony that I have heard in such a short period of time that has made a more dramatic impact on me. I want to thank all of you for your courage."[32]

The press coverage of dialysis stories was generally positive and upbeat, focusing on the patients who were gainfully employed and doing well. "A Kidney Patient Can Live Normally," was a typical headline; and the text explained how one lawyer brought his secretary to the treatment center and caught up on his dictation and telephone calls while on dialysis. Another patient, a truck driver, scheduled his treatments around his regular runs.[33] An account in *Newsweek* of the technology featured a photograph of a patient playing tennis and eating (however improbable) "high off the hog." A *New York Times* story about the Gottsho Foundation (which donated dialysis machines to hospitals and individual patients) noted that during dialysis "the patient is free to read, watch television, study, knit or do paper work."[34] Qualifications to the effect that some but not all patients were able to perform such feats did not often appear in the stories.

Occasionally, the darker side slipped through. Carl Salamensky was one patient who could not tolerate life on dialysis. Not only a bland diet and incessant itching but persistent sleeplessness and headaches drove him to the point of declaring, as the *Newsweek* headline put it, "I Can't Take Any More." Still, his agony probably would not have attracted press coverage except for the fact that Salamensky was so desperate for a kidney transplant that he took out an advertisement ("Urgently Wanted Kidney") and offered to pay $3000 to the next of kin for a cadaveric donation. It was the advertisement that was newsworthy, not the pain and suffering.[35]

For all the rhetorical commitment to elevating life over money, it was still necessary to estimate costs for dialysis and to determine, or at least arguably contend, that the national bill for ESRD would be affordable. As it turned out, this assignment became relatively routine, not because the facts were clear but precisely because they were not. It was exceedingly difficult for Congress, or even for the Bureau of the Budget, to predict with any accuracy the demand for a novel medical treatment—just as it would later be difficult to predict the demand for medical services under a national health insurance system. Washington officials, particularly in the early 1970s, had to trust more to outside expert opinion—but the experts in the technology were also the advocates for the technology. In effect, the proponents of the intervention got to define its probabilities and expenses. Although critics would later charge that Congress had misled the country and had not done its homework ("Medicarelessness," the *New York Times* called it), the number of uncertainties was so great that one can sympathize with advocates' predilection to keep estimates of expenditures low, and congressional readiness to accept their figures.

Before calculating the present and future costs of reimbursing dialysis expenses for all patients, it was first necessary to estimate the number of patients who would require the intervention. Arriving at this figure, however, was a function not only of the epidemiology of end-stage renal disease in the general population and the prevailing rates of mortality (whether on or not on dialysis) but also of how many patients would opt to undergo kidney transplantation instead of dialysis and how many would have access to an organ. (The experts assumed that more rather than fewer patients would take advantage of the transplant procedure, thereby incurring a one-time fixed cost, and reducing the overall costs of a reimbursement program.) At the same time, cost estimates had to calculate the number of patients who would use home dialysis, which was cheaper than hospital dialysis, at least in the long term. And the estimates also had to take into account changing criteria for receiving dialysis: such negative indicators as very advanced age, co-morbid disease, disabling psychiatric factors, and other potentially limiting conditions might not be so compelling once the technology became more available and the techniques more advanced.

The most educated guesses were that somewhere around 10,000 patients in 1972 needed dialysis, but that number was anything but hard and fixed and seems to have been taken from the 1967 estimates of the Gottschalk committee, which were made well before knowledge of the technology had spread through medical and lay circles. It was ever so convenient to keep repeating the same, and in retrospect far too low, number, and to miss all the considerations that went into the fact that, 20 years later, there would be not 10,000 but 150,000 patients on dialysis.

Moreover, to gauge costs accurately, it was necessary to set a price on the technology, and advocates were not being unreasonable in anticipating a decline in price for the machines over time. After all, kidney transplantation costs already had dropped by one-third; and the prices for computers and other electronic equipment typically fell by as much as 50% within a few years of a product's introduction.

Still other contingencies had to be evaluated. As advocates reminded Congress, it was also expensive to die of uremia. And surely it was appropriate to factor into the calculations the fact that seemingly all, or mostly all, patients on dialysis would be earning a living, paying taxes, supporting their families, and thus making returns on the investment in technology. Better to pay for the machine than to pay for the welfare costs while patients sat home waiting to die. By the time all the possible variables were brought together, a final price tag of $250 million for dialysis seemed about right. That the figure turned out, first, to be too low by a factor of 4 and then, a few years later, by a factor of 12 was not anticipated by anyone.

One final consideration reduced the attention paid to the costs of dialysis, and that was a hope (for some, a conviction) that federal support for dialysis would be the proverbial first step to national health insurance. There was less reason to fret about costs when sooner rather than later dialysis would be folded into a general insurance scheme. Advocacy groups took pains to merge their own narrower concern with national health insurance. The NAPH newsletters frequently urged members to write Congress in support of "the creation of a universal health insurance plan." Indeed, it stated confidently: "A fundamental change in the organization of the nation's health care programs is imminent. All signs point to a unification . . . into a single large unit. . . . It should result in cheaper and better health care not only for dialysis patients but for everyone."[36] Dr. George Schreiner of the National Kidney Association reiterated these sentiments: "I hope that, eventually, a national medical care system of some kind will include catastrophic illness provisions which can deal effectively with this problem, as with other catastrophic illnesses."[37] Or as Dr. William J. Flanigan, representing the National Kidney Foundation, put it: "We think in the case of chronic kidney patients the need [for federal coverage] is pressing and immediate," and should be a "first step toward a national health insurance plan."[38] In sum, whatever the costs of dialysis, they paled by comparison with the costs of national health insurance and, therefore, ought not to be a barrier to implementation.

Linking dialysis with national health insurance had the critical advantage of explaining why dialysis patients should be given preferential treatment over other patient groups. At the close of debate on the 1972 act, one senator, objecting to the funding bill, asked why dialysis patients should receive such a windfall when others with equally grave and expensive medical needs were ignored: "There is the problem of the hemophiliacs, who must constantly receive blood transfusions if they are to remain alive. Nobody is worried about them in this bill. This demonstrates that we are picking out one particular sector of the whole health care problem, and because it is dramatic, we are trying to push it ahead of everything else."[39] The short answer to his question was that national health insurance would eventually cover these other conditions as well. The long answer involved all the considerations we have addressed here. In the 1970s, dialysis patients received preferential treatment because of the power of technology creep, middle-class advocacy, American attitudes toward life-saving machines, and a political process which, when the case was framed specifically and dramatically, elevated life over money.

Unlike the iron lung, dialysis policy soon generated a backlash, not simply because the promise of national health insurance went unrealized but because the program itself violated almost all of the original expectations. As the machines became more widely available and cost became irrelevant, the criteria for dialysis grew more relaxed. Dialysis patients were soon considerably older, sicker, and poorer than they had been before. When the program began, the median age of the patients was 46; 15 years later, it had climbed to 61. The percentage of those on dialysis who were above the age of 65 increased from one-quarter to over one-third. At the same time, more patients had other grave health problems. In the 1970s, less than 15% of dialysis patients had chronic diabetes; in the 1980s, the percentage swelled to 24%. So, too, the program lost its white and middle class character. In the late 1960s, only 10% of dialysis patients were black; in 1990, 29% were black. Perhaps most important in fueling the ESRD controversy, total expenses were four times greater than had been predicted, mostly because the number of people who received benefits expanded so dramatically. In 1973, the program served 10,000 patients at a cost of $229 million. By 1990, it was serving 150,000 patients at a cost of $3 billion.[40] In sum, a program that was to spend a trivial amount so as to allow a relatively small number of healthy young professionals to go back to work was suddenly now spending billions to keep alive thousands of decrepit elderly.

This transformation could have been interpreted in very favorable terms. Indeed, some observers were delighted that dialysis techniques and physician skills and experience had become so refined that older and sicker patients could be treated. By the same token, the fact that patients were poorer and blacker provided ample justification for the federal intervention;

without it, the disparities in health care would have continued to be great, and minorities would have suffered unnecessary deaths. In effect, the rising cost testified to rising eligibility, for which Americans should be proud.

Nevertheless, these same facts generated a number of criticisms of the ESRD program, the most notable of which was the 1984 book by Henry Aaron and William Schwartz, *The Painful Prescription: Rationing Health Care.* Their argument was very sophisticated and nuanced (which would not be characteristic, as we shall see, of much of the later literature); it invoked the ESRD program as a consummate, albeit not exclusive, example of the problems that were confronting American health policy. Comparing U. S. to British practices, Aaron and Schwartz reported that 230 per million Americans were undergoing dialysis, compared to 69 per million British. The striking difference reflected not a higher incidence of disease but an unwillingness in the United States to limit access to the technology. Unlike the British, Americans did not keep patients off the machine because of age or other accompanying diseases. The root causes for this distinction were not hard to identify. In England, the National Health Service had to provide care to an entire population from one budget and it was loath to devote a disproportionate share of its resources to dialysis; moreover, it was under almost no political or legal pressure to do so. In the United States, without national health insurance but with well-organized patient advocacy groups and malpractice lawyers, resource allocation decisions were made on an ad hoc basis, meeting the costs of one disease but not another.

Aaron and Schwartz were convinced that the time was fast approaching when Americans, too, would have to accept budget constraints. Given escalating costs, with ESRD as a prime example, Americans would be forced to rethink a policy that used "technologically sophisticated and costly methods to provide medical care that is sometimes of slight value," and often served to reduce "the quality of the dying patient's remaining life." In their view, unless Americans restrained expenditures, they would "suffer a continual increase in medical expenditures and in expenditures yielding benefits worth less than the costs." But of course, as Aaron and Schwartz concluded, to ration the use of medical machines would inevitably be, in the terms of their title, "painful."[41]

Just how painful? And how controversial? One need only read a 1991 *New York Times* Op-Ed contribution by Richard Margolis, himself a journalist and a dialysis patient, to appreciate the dimensions. Alert to the controversies spawned by dialysis, Margolis based his case for the machine by contrasting American expenditures for the Gulf War with its expenditures for ESRD. A country that spent billions of dollars to bring about death could surely afford $3 billion a year to give life. "Watching life's elixir trickle into my body," Margolis wrote, "I wish for a world in which our errands of mercy were as ardently admired as our sorties of destruction."[42] If for Senator Hartke in 1972 the telling comparison was to the annual costs for cosmetics, for Margolis it was the costs for a military campaign. Obviously, proponents of dialysis, or any other medical life-saving technology for that matter, had no difficulty in devising persuasive comparisons for justifying government support. Which was precisely why the American Way in health care seemed to be in trouble.

5 Rationing the Respirator

The challenge that dialysis in the late 1970s and 1980s posed for traditional American attitudes and policies toward life-saving technologies soon emerged in still more acute form around the artificial ventilator, more popularly known as the respirator. By the early 1990s, the pressing question had become how to establish boundaries around the use of the machine, not how to maximize its availability. A significant cadre of health economists, health care administrators, and, more surprisingly, bioethicists and physicians were concluding that the goal of policy should not be to provide patients with full and ready access to medical technologies but to circumscribe access to these technologies. And it appeared, at least insofar as the respirator was concerned, that the general public agreed with this approach. The driving question had become how to say no to technology.

The new critics went well beyond Aaron and Schwartz in designing detailed blueprints for limiting access to advanced medical technologies. For some of them, the goal was to save taxpayers' dollars; for others it was to make funds available for a national health insurance program. For still others it was the occasion to try to bring new dimensions of spirituality to American life and the American way of death. But whatever their purpose, the arguments they presented all gave the idea of restraint, or in the term of the day, rationing, an unprecedented centrality and a moral legitimacy in policy thinking and policy initiatives.

Unlike the iron lung or the dialysis machine, the artificial ventilator was not the invention of a single individual. The machine evolved, slowly and fitfully, over almost three-quarters of a century. The iron lung actually played only a minor part in its history. The first of the breathing machines had worked by creating a zone of negative pressure around the diaphragm and chest; by contrast, its successor applied positive pressure. The respirator forced air directly into the lungs and filled them at a rate set by the machine, independent of any lung mechanics or for that matter any reflexive activity by the brain's breathing center. In fact, a major impetus to the development of the respirator was the cumbersome and unwieldy character of the iron lung itself; not only was the machine large and noisy, but caring for a patient within it, washing him or suctioning out phlegm, was tedious and exhausting. A second and even more important consideration was that the iron lung could not meet the novel demands of a new generation of highly skilled and aggressive heart and lung surgeons. They were technically capable of operating directly on these vital organs, provided that some means were available for maintaining patients' respiratory functioning during and immediately after the surgery.

The challenge was met because of a series of advances, oftentimes unrelated, in disparate fields. The respirator drew on knowledge of lung physiology first acquired in World War II to meet the needs of submarine personnel traveling beneath the ocean and airforce personnel flying at high altitudes. A new understanding of blood gases and the ability to measure them that developed in the 1950s made it possible to monitor the effects of ventilation on patients. No less important, the respirator drew heavily on the experience in Copenhagen in 1952, when an epidemic of polio broke out and hundreds of patients suddenly needed respiratory assistance. With iron lungs in very short supply (no NFIP operated in Denmark), physicians, in desperation, turned to positive pressure ventilation, at first relying on medical students to supply it by hand and, later, rigging up mechanical means to accomplish the task.

As these disparate developments came together, physicians recognized the usefulness of mechanically applied positive pressure to treat patients suffering from respiratory deficiencies due to illness or surgical interventions. With time and experience, they expanded the indications for artificial respiration and improved the rates of success. Thus Massachusetts General Hospital in 1958 ventilated a total of 66 patients for 24 hours or more. Ten years later it was ventilating almost 900 patients, and by 1982, some 2000. All the while, survival rates climbed to about 75%.

In this way, an efficient, convenient, mobile, and effective ventilator took its place at the bedside and in the operating room. The machine took over the breathing function for patients with a temporary loss of pulmonary function (because of surgery, an asthma attack, pulmonary edema, or drug overdose), or with a more permanent loss of lung or brain function. In either case, it had the capability of maintaining the patient's respiration not just for hours or days, but for months and years. The ventilator also sparked the most significant organizational change in the contemporary hospital. Into the 1950s, critically ill hospital patients had been treated on the general wards, moved perhaps to the front beds near the nursing stations, but not to special units. By 1970, every tertiary medical center and many community hospitals had intensive care units (ICUs), in which the great majority of patients were on respirators.[1]

Not surprisingly, therefore, the respirator, like the iron lung and dialysis machine before it, was initially celebrated for ushering in a new era in medical care. The technology received due credit for the success of new forms of cardio-thoracic surgery; without it, surgeons would not have been able to graft onto the heart new coronary arteries to replace clogged vessels. So, too, everyone appreciated that artificial ventilators kept patients with pneumonia or other lung dysfunctions alive so that antibiotics had the time to work their cure. The respirator was also understood to be the essential technology in the ICU—the two are so inseparable that in most hospitals, a patient cannot be on a respirator without being in an ICU. Indeed, enthusiasm for the respirator in the ICU was so unbounded that the efficacy of the units was never tested by clinical trials. No sooner was the technology available than it was implemented; it seemed unethical (in the United States, although not in England) to conduct randomized trials, wherein some patients went to an ICU while others remained on the ward, and their outcomes were compared. The presumption was that intensive care produced better results, in large measure due to the marvels of the breathing machine.

All this ardor notwithstanding, the respirator, in relatively short order and even more notably than the iron lung or dialysis machine, provoked a hostile response from segments of both the medical profession and the general public. As astonishing as the machine's capabilities were, it assumed the aura of a profoundly "unnatural" device, mostly because of its ability to keep alive for long periods of time people who were in the last stages of advanced disease, in a vegetative state, or actually brain dead. The marvels that the respirator accomplished in the operating room were often glossed over, in the sense that commentators did not regularly associate this technology with extraordinary surgical feats. Accounts of open heart surgery, for example, focused more on the surgeon than on the equipment. At the same time, stories began circulating about the compulsory "thirty thousand dollar funeral," that is, the cost of keeping Uncle Timothy alive on the respirator for a couple of weeks before he was finally allowed to die. The ICU became Atlanta—one could no more get to a southern city without stopping off in Atlanta than get to heaven without stopping off in the ICU.

One of the first expressions of this negative sentiment appeared in response to a report of the M. D. Anderson Hospital in Houston, Texas, an outstanding cancer treatment center. Of the 180 cancer patients it had put on respirators between 1975 and 1977, only 26% could be successfully weaned from the machines, and only 7% were alive six months later. Drawing on this experience, one physician and historian of mechanical ventilation concluded: "Mechanical ventilation had joined renal dialysis . . . as technologies that could prolong life at a vegetative level . . . where restoration to a functional level sufficient to permit the independent carrying out of activities of daily living was by no means assured."[2]

The skepticism about the technology also stemmed from the average age of patients sustained for long periods of time on respirators. The iron lung had served those under 30, the dialysis machine, at least at first, those under 45. The majority of respirator-dependent patients, however, were well over 65. Moreover, with the iron lung and initially with dialysis, rates of recovery increased over time, making it easier to justify these interventions in terms of subsequent quality of life. But putting someone on a respirator too often seemed a futile intervention, serving merely to postpone an inevitable funeral.

The starkest images of the respirator, however, were transmitted to the entire nation through the case of Karen Ann Quinlan, heretofore unknown but destined to become arguably the most famous patient in American medicine. Quinlan was the headline story that taught Americans about the respirator the way Frederic Snite's odyssey taught them about the iron lung. The chief component of the Quinlan lesson, however, was that health care providers, left to themselves, would foist a machine on patients and on families who wanted no part of it. For the first time, a medical machine and its keepers appeared inhumane, even tyrannical. Nowhere in the iron lung literature and only sporadically in the dialysis literature was the theme of how to avoid the machine as prominent as it was with the respirator. This was technology as enemy.

The Karen Ann Quinlan story is so well known as to require only a brief synopsis. On the night of April 15, 1975, she was brought to a New Jersey hospital emergency room in a coma whose etiology was never fully explained and from which she never emerged. After several months of hoping against hope, her parents recognized that she would not recover, and they requested St. Clair's Hospital to remove her from the respirator that had been controlling her breathing. The Quinlans, who were practicing Catholics and had sought church guidance, were told by their priest that respirator care was "extraordinary." Returning Karen to her "natural state," that is, taking her off the machine, even if she were to die, was a morally correct action. But the hospital refused a request for removal that the family, their religious leaders, and, later, most of the public thought was reasonable and appropriate. The Quinlans petitioned the Superior Court of New Jersey for relief and when this lower court turned them down, they took the case to the state Supreme Court, which ruled in their favor. After another two months of wrangling with the hospital and the doctors, Karen was "weaned" from the respirator, transferred to a long-term care facility, and despite predictions of imminent death, survived, off the respirator, for another nine years.[3]

The Quinlan saga taught Americans how oppressive a medical machine might be. The Quinlan family never permitted photographs of Karen Ann (despite lucrative offers from some newspapers), but there were numerous descriptions of how she lay curled in fetal position, periodically emitting low, dull groans. It would be hard to imagine a more compelling case of a technology performing the most unnatural of functions. Courtesy of the iron lung, Snite had traveled round the world; courtesy of dialysis, Shep Glaser was carrying on a vigorous life as an advocate. But courtesy of the respirator, Karen Ann Quinlan lay trapped in a twilight zone between life and death.

As a result of the massive publicity generated by the case, a growing number of Americans began instructing relatives and doctors—formally in living wills and proxy appointments or informally in conversation—how they wished to be treated should they ever be in Quinlan's condition. In this way, the machine became identified with the need for patients to control end-of-life decisions so as to make certain that they would not be victims of the technology. Indeed, as courts became more meticulous about the type of evidence required before allowing hospitals to terminate respirator treatment for incompetent patients (insisting upon written and formal expressions of preferences), state legislatures responded by enacting codes that legalized a variety of mechanisms to promote advance decision making. Following on a U. S. Supreme Court decision upholding a rigorous evidentiary standard for establishing prior expressions of patients' wishes, New York State enacted a health proxy act which required hospitals to ask all patients upon admission whether they had appointed a proxy, and in the event that they had not, to supply them with the forms to do so. In this way, the reasoning went, a patient's personal preferences might be able to trump the reflexive response of physicians and hospitals to use, whatever the patient's condition or prognosis, a respirator.

Thus, setting down end-of-life instructions emerged as the primary strategy for avoiding the potentially appalling consequences of medical technology. That the strategy was generally ineffective (which is even more apparent now than it was then) is not nearly as interesting as the fact that it reflected an unusually dark vision of medical technology. The impulse (here attributed to physicians) to overuse the machine had to be thwarted—a dictum that may not sound especially surprising in terms of the respirator, but certainly was unprecedented in terms of the history of life-saving medical devices.

Part of the revulsion against the respirator involved a sense of dignity and decency—that was no way to die—but part of it also reflected considerations of cost. Earlier complaints about $30,000 funerals turned into bitter objections from numerous hospital administrators, state and federal budget directors, and families, about $100,000 funerals. It became fashionable to suggest, with more fervor than data, that escalating health care costs could be contained if only patients made end-of-life decisions. Living wills and proxy appointments, which had originally been conceived as ways to enhance patient autonomy, were being heralded as the solution to escalating health care expenditures. The thinking was that patients who defined in advance what treatments they would or would not undergo in the event of serious illness would be eager to forgo respirator care and thus die more cheaply. The goal was not so much to promote choice as to serve a collective good. Refusing to go on the machine was emerging as a new social duty.

Alert to this shift in attitude, a number of commentators came to believe that the American public was finally prepared to deal realistically with medical technologies. Because of the machine's capabilities (to keep the dead alive) and accompanying costs (thousands of dollars a day), public policy seemed primed for tough talk and hard choices. Although never articulated quite this bluntly, this vision influenced numerous policy analysts and public officials. The hostility to the respirator was interpreted to represent hostility to medical technology more generally. Rationing was on the way to becoming acceptable.

Just how widespread this perspective became, and how much validity it enjoyed, emerges not simply from the writings of economists but from a quarter that one would have presumed to be least hospitable to this type of approach, that is, bioethicists. The field, born in the 1960s, was originally dedicated to the advancement of individual rights. The enemy was paternalism, whether exercised by the physician or the state, and the goal was to enlarge autonomy. To this end, bioethicists led the movement to promote informed consent and to compel doctors to be truthful in relating a grim diagnosis. But in the late 1980s and early 1990s, some of them entered the rationing debate and shifted their advocacy from individual rights to collective needs. American health care programs, insisted Daniel Callahan, president of the prestigious and influential Hastings Center, should be "fostering the common good and collective health of society, not the particularized good of individuals." This transformation gave a powerful aura of legitimacy to the rationing discussions, and suggested that painful choices might well be acceptable to a broader public. Apparently there were ethically appropriate criteria that could be invoked to exclude patients from the machine, regardless of their own personal feelings. Whatever one thinks of the intellectual exercise, the very readiness to frame the issue in these terms encouraged and reinforced a major shift in health policy.

The most prominent and active bioethicist spreading this message was Callahan, not only in several books but in many public speeches and television appearances. Although the specifics of his position shifted over time, he steadfastly argued in favor of rationing medicine. His first target was the treatment of the very old. Once people reach ripe old age (the age is not specified but Callahan hints that the late 70s would be about right), they would be entitled to comfort and nursing care but not to high-tech, machine-driven medical services. Whatever their wishes, their doctor's judgment, or their children's desires, the constraint would hold. They might be healthy and wise, perhaps only requiring a respirator to tide them over for a few days while they recovered from an acute illness, but if they had passed over the age divide, they would not have access to the technology.

Callahan advanced a variety of justifications for his position, each of them having some support in the larger community. At times, he contended that such a restrictive policy is what the aged already want—as witness the eagerness to stay off respirators at the end of life. At other times, he argued that these restrictions are what the aged "should want," which is, after all, quite different and notably paternalistic. At some points, Callahan played the role of health care economist, worried about the growing cost of medical care and the percentage of national resources devoted to health; at other points he joined advocates for national health insurance, trying to reduce costs so as to facilitate its implementation. Then at still other points he was a social theorist, speculating about the conflict for resources between the generations or arguing that it is time for 1960s individual-istic values to give way to community values. Finally, he appeared as an old-fashioned pulpit moralist, seeking to infuse a new meaning in old age and death.

Whatever conceptual confusions were bred by this scattershot approach, one unifying theme invoked by Callahan, and others as well, was an almost naive appeal to the concept of the "natural." The enemy became "modern-ism," which turned out to be a characterization, really a caricature, of tradi-tional American values. Modernism in Callahan's terms was the "belief that human ingenuity can bring about a better future . . . that nature is not fixed or normative in its ends but is malleable to human purposes and construc-tion." In medicine, the core of "the modernizing project is an attempt to deny limits, to act as if old age can do without them, or could proceed by pretending they do not exist." This modernism represented a denial of the "whole of life," of the fact "that life has relatively fixed stages," and that "old age is of necessity marked by decline . . . [and] death may present an abso-lute limit." He then proposed a definition of a "natural life span," that is, the period when one's life possibilities have been realized, when one has discharged moral obligations to others, and when death "will not seem to others an offense to sense or sensibility." All of this led him to conclude that medicine "should be used not for the further extension of life of the aged, but only for the full achievement of a natural and fitting life span."[4]

Callahan became almost rhapsodic about the good that this exercise in rationing could accomplish, celebrating it as the occasion to rethink not only the place of medicine in our lives but the fundamental purposes of our lives. "The financial crisis facing the healthcare system provides a superb, if probably painful, occasion to ask some basic questions once again about health and human life." The American value system apparently got it all so very wrong that limitations, however painful to apply, become positively "superb" occasions for finally getting it right.

Because Americans coveted every technological fix to ward off disease and death, no matter how scarce or expensive, Callahan insisted that only a formal rationing system could curb so insatiable an appetite. When the driving force was individual demand, efforts to make health care delivery more efficient or to devise new reimbursement formulas to contain hospital and physician reimbursement or to improve technology assessment would not resolve the predicament. The only effective solution was to devise criteria that would limit individual treatment and then follow, really impose, them. And the criteria? We should provide that much health care that maintains in good working order the political and legal system, the national defense, the pursuit and transmission of knowledge and culture, and the familial and philanthropic institutions that bind the society. Precisely because individual demand was boundless, mounting medical costs were swallowing up resources needed to meet other pressing social needs. Thus instead of underwriting more medical research to produce more advanced medical technologies, government should be investing in schools, industrial development, highways, parks, and recreation. "Time," warned Callahan, "is running out on the expansive, and expensive, enterprise of contemporary medicine." After all, despite some exceptions, the "average level of individual and societal health is *already* adequate to meet general needs. . . . Whatever the shortcomings of our social institutions, the poor health of their participants is not the cause." With his eye on Detroit, not the National Institutes of Health, Callahan asked: "Has anyone ever seriously suggested that poor health is the reason we no longer compete well with the Japanese?"[5]

Within medicine, Callahan would reverse inherited priorities and fund care and prevention, not cure. Programs should serve first the chronic patient who needs social services (hospice, nursing, and institutional care), not the acute patient who needs high technology interventions. He also favored preventive medicine and prenatal care, along with low-tech, low cost, and effective interventions such as the delivery of antibiotics and simple emergency medicine. These procedures addressed the "common threat to all," and ensured the "adequate functioning of social institutions." What should be eliminated? Dialysis, of course, and intensive care to the elderly. These expensive interventions merely solve "individualized problems" and yield a low quality of life.[6]

Although these arguments have glaring weaknesses, they did not stop him, or others, from giving rationing a newfound respectability. Take, for example, Callahan's standard of providing only that health care which the community requires for its good order. Even before the advent of curative medicine (which is no more than 50 years old), many societies managed to achieve an "adequate functioning of social institutions." In Europe, premodern plagues aside, health was rarely the determining consideration in maintaining social stability; in the United States, at least from the eighteenth century on, the poor health of some segments of our citizenry has rarely been associated with social disorder. In other words, however appealing it may be to suggest that community stability and well-being are the criteria against which to judge medical interventions, they really do little service in distinguishing what kind of medicine the public should have.

There was an even more notable flaw in the Callahan presentation, and one that had the most significant implications for the entire effort to make rationing seem equitable. Callahan had a secret that he did not divulge until his arguments were almost concluded. Then we suddenly learned that rationing health care and restricting individual choice is to affect only *public* programs. Individuals should be able to receive all the technology and services that they can afford to pay for; only government-funded programs must elevate care over cure, and refuse dialysis and respirators to the elderly. The private sector was free to satisfy every individual demand for technological medicine.

Conceding that his plan was "not too different from the system we now have in a crude form," Callahan offered one central defense for the different standards. Were the public sector to ration high-tech medicine, the government would have the funds to implement national health insurance. A frankly two-tier medical system would improve the access of the poor to general medical services. But would the poor, particularly the elderly poor, and their advocates, be content with this smaller package? Callahan believed they would be if they understood that health care is not an end, that communitarian ideals are critical, and that health care costs must be contained. These three principles would be able "to overcome the animus of so many egalitarians against anything other than one-tier medicine."[7] Thus what began as a sermon closed with an endorsement of market-driven inequalities. Rationing became the fate awaiting the poor, not the middle classes. In the end, Jeremiah embraced Herbert Spencer.

The enthusiasm that marked Callahan's approach characterized the work of a number of other bioethicists as well. They, too, shared an eagerness to help make hard choices. To be sure, their designs were flawed and they were far too ready to accept marked degrees of inequity. But the message that they disseminated was that placing limits on the delivery of health care was ethically sound and, therefore, if carried out shrewdly, politically acceptable.

This was certainly the thrust of the arguments presented by John Kilner in *Who Lives? Who Dies?* and by Paul Menzel in *Strong Medicine*. Both of them took inherited American attitudes toward life-saving medical technologies, particularly toward dialysis, as their negative reference point. To Kilner, it was nothing more than a "popular myth" that Americans had sufficient resources to guarantee access for everyone to all medical technologies.[8] Menzel posited an even broader but no less inescapable conflict between the well-being of the individual patient and the social drive for "economic efficiency," which could not be satisfied merely by eliminating waste. Both were ready to issue painful prescriptions, which in their terms would be "strong medicine to swallow."[9]

Kilner, focusing on the micro issues, laid out an exhaustive catalogue of the principles that have been suggested or used to give one patient rather than another access to a limited resource. He identified no less than 16 criteria, divided into social, medical, and personal categories, ranging from social worth (as per the Seattle committee) and favored group (nationals ought to receive benefits before foreigners), to imminent death (the dying patient should have priority over the very sick), age, the ability to pay, and first-come, first-served. Kilner outlined the justifications and weaknesses of each principle and possible grounds of agreement. The exercise was so schematic as to be altogether mechanical, but in his schema, many different principles enjoyed some degree of legitimacy. In fact, Kilner was far more eager to identify winning arguments than to cast doubt on the wisdom of the entire rationing enterprise.

Whatever the difficulties of choosing among criteria, Kilner confidently proposed his own rationing formula: give priority to persons facing imminent death; to those with "special responsibilities" to family or community; and to those who would use less of a scarce resource than others so as to maximize the number who can be treated. To distribute the remaining resources, he advocated a lottery.[10] These rankings, however, reflect little more than his personal preferences. We never learn why priorities should be given to the dying (at any age?) or to those with family responsibilities (are we back to the middle-class bias of the who-shall-live committees?). Still, his underlying message is clear: although the exercise of rationing is complicated, it is the right thing to do.

Paul Menzel was even more prepared to defend the proposition that "a cautious but courageous rationing of care" can be legitimate without having "to wait for people to sign on some dotted line." One may rightly presume a patient's consent when a societal consensus existed on the validity of the action, where the action would bring important gains, and where obtaining actual consent would be "impossible or prohibitively costly." With less caution than Aaron and Schwartz, he embraced the British model in dialysis—let physicians simply tell ESRD patients that nothing can be done for them. Although Menzel was troubled by the fact that physicians masked the reasons for their decision—making it appear that the disease, not the allocation of resources by the National Health Service was the root of the problem—he doggedly insisted that such rationing was in accord with prior consent. "As a voter, the patient probably supported the government's policy—at least before his kidney failed, and in any case he supports the political procedures by which those decisions are made." The physician was, therefore, obliged to respect this apparent prior consent: "Would she not be insulting him as an average British citizen proud of his NHS if she ignored scarcity criteria and got him on dialysis?"[11] But then why did doctors find it necessary to obfuscate the message if such a degree of prior agreement actually existed?

Menzel also advanced a "duty to die cheaply." To forgo the use of scarce and expensive medical resources to combat terminal illness was not only noble and heroic, but "allowing oneself to die to save resources can be one's moral duty." Moreover, this duty was socially enforceable, that is, governments may compel people to die cheaply. In defense of this proposition, Menzel invoked the language of Christian ethics. Not to die cheaply was to pursue "our own vanity," to make "idols out of ourselves," to elevate egoism over communal obligations, and to reject the sovereignty of God. So persuaded was he of the force of these principles that he extended the duty to die cheaply from patients with terminal illness to those who needed "quasi-terminal care," those who would receive a few years more of low quality life, and those who were "severely demented." "Life-extending care of the severely demented becomes a first-order candidate for restrictions if we take seriously the task of matching rationing policies with people's actual values." How can we be certain that these policies represent people's values? Because among the over-65 population, a "significant number of patients themselves reject dialysis." As for those with severe dementia, the conclusion to withhold care was "virtually unquestionable."[12]

Dimly aware of the potential mischief that such policies might well bring, Menzel maintained that "prior consent does not give a simple green light to any and all efficient policies." But he was incapable of explaining how or why an impulse to economize would be checked. Instead, he presumed that the consensus he discerned would always be equitably implemented and such an exercise of collective authority was warranted. He did not pause before the possibility that minorities often need protection against majorities, that a program that denies the severely demented access to treatment may come to include the severely retarded or the chronic schizophrenic. In all, he lacked any appreciation of the prospect that when the medicine gets strong enough, the other fellow may be forced to swallow it.

How to understand such narrowness of vision and conceptual inadequacy among these bioethicists?[13] The answer rests, in part, on their commitment to serve societal ends; the community had replaced the individual in the hierarchy of values. But in part, too, these arguments presumed that the use of medical technology had changed in a way that undermined the desirability of sustaining the original American commitment to open access. As exemplified by the dialysis machine and the respirator, one would not necessarily want to be rescued by medicine. Indeed, it is impossible to imagine anyone, let alone a bioethicist, living in the shadow of the Holocaust, advocating a rationing system that sacrificed the "severely demented" unless medical technology had lost some or much of its glamour and attraction. In this sense, the respirator and the dialysis machine came to exemplify advanced technologies. The rationing literature more frequently invoked the use of these two machines than any other interventions. As we shall see, this focus distorted the ethical issues and misread public attitudes. But for a while it seemed that rationing was not only right but palatable. People would fill the painful prescriptions and take the strong medicine.

Not only bioethicists but a cadre of physicians helped to make arguments in favor of rationing creditable. True, the great majority of doctors who wrote about scarce resources insisted that medicine's exclusive commitment had to be to the well-being of the individual patient. But a sizable, even influential, minority parted company and tried to make rationing consistent with the Hippocratic Oath.

Take, for example, the argument advanced by Troyen Brennan, a physician and lawyer on the faculty of Harvard. He, too, espoused the need to ration: "There must be limits on the resources we as a society put into health care." To be sure, physicians at the bedside were not the ones to decide which lives should be saved and which should not. Rather, "Physician decisions should be made within guidelines developed by broad social consensus" so that "cost controls work in the best possible manner." This principle presented, Brennan said very little about the substance of the guidelines. He was adept at identifying what doctors should not do. As against the British experience with dialysis, he did not want them misleading patients. Moreover, as against Callahan, he did not want rationing to be arbitrary—not all

80-year-olds are alike. He worried, too, about the consequences of letting the wealthier classes buy out of the system. If an ability to pay becomes the determining principle, "the poor will likely bear the brunt of rationing." But rather than abandon the quest for the holy grail of a fair rationing system or conclude that the obstacles are simply too great to overcome, Brennan ended on a very different note: rationing could be equitable and physicians should help achieve it—even though he was incapable of giving specificity to these general propositions.[14]

A lack of specificity was certainly not the problem with Dr. William Knaus's approach to rationing. The George Washington University medical school professor devised a formula which he sells as a computer program under the title Apache. It is a mathematically derived weighing of patient characteristics in ICU settings that attempts to predict who will or will not survive. Thus, a patient who is over 85 years of age, with a high score on the acute physiology scale, a diagnosis of leukemia or lymphoma, who had been in the hospital immediately before entering the unit, carries a diagnosis of sepsis or cardiac arrest, and has already been in the unit for 31 days or more, has, according to the Apache scale, a 90% likelihood of dying in the ICU, regardless of what physicians do.

Knaus's scale has obvious value as a research tool, allowing investigators to measure which interventions raise or lower the odds of survival. It is useful, too, for quality control, identifying ICUs, for example, that have better or worse survival rates. It may also help to answer questions from patients and their families about prognosis; a physician asked about the odds of survival has a ready answer. But the critical concern for Knaus was whether such a formula, even improved to the point where it has 95% accuracy, might be used to limit treatment. Was this a tool that would fulfill the goal of curbing medical care at the end of life, or for that matter, at any point in life? In cases where the patient score is, say, 95, would Blue Cross or Medicare be entitled to deny reimbursement for ICU care?

Knaus was by no means unhappy with such a prospect. "If our technical ability to provide intensive care expands while our financial capabilities become more restricted, the capability of evaluating competing patients' requirements or their abilities to benefit from intensive care could become more important." In other words, an exercise in rationing would be justified provided it rested on complete and accurate data. There was nothing wrong with the policy, only with the existing power of the measurement.[15]

Just how dubious the ethics of such decision making would be becomes apparent if one invokes the standards of criminal justice. There might well exist a 90% likelihood that an unemployed, drug-using, 21-year-old with a long criminal record and no known family has a 90% likelihood of committing a crime within the next twelve months. Yet to incarcerate such a person before he committed a crime on the basis of a predictive scale would violate shared ideas on fairness. Moreover, better that nine guilty men go free than one innocent man be wrongfully punished—a formula that puts a different frame around 90% reliability. Bringing this orientation directly into medicine would mean that it was far better that nine patients receive futile treatment than one patient dies needlessly. But this represented the very kind of reasoning that Knaus was opposing. For him, an acceptable and fair rationing system only awaited the derivation of more powerful formulas.

The most elusive but intriguing evidence of how far Americans seemed to be ready to go in saying no to medical technologies like the respirator emerged from several popular and well-received narrative accounts of care at the end of life. Philip Roth's *Patrimony* and Andrew Malcolm's *Someday*, along with the spectacular sales of a self-help book on suicide, *Final Exit*, all suggested that officials could start rationing medical treatment without incurring popular wrath.

As described in *Patrimony*, Herman Roth, Philip's 86-year-old father, learned that he had a nonmalignant tumor pressing against the brain stem, which could be excised by surgery. Although the surgery had a 75% survival rate (and undoubtedly would have been paid for by Medicare), it required, depending on which surgeon you talked to, either one eight- to ten-hour procedure or two seven- to eight-hour procedures several months apart. The recuperation period would be several months long, and Mr. Roth would have to learn how to walk again. The surgeons he and Philip consulted were certainly prepared to do the procedure, and they had no doubt that the alternative, to do nothing, was far worse. But Mr. Roth, with his family's concurrence, declined the operation. Philip discussed other treatment options with his father, who then signed a living will declaring that were he to become incompetent, he did not want "mechanical respiration when I am no longer able to sustain my own breathing."

Despite some real misgivings, Philip respected these wishes at the decisive moment:

> Early on the morning of his death, when I arrived at the hospital emergency room . . . I was confronted by an attending physician prepared to take 'extraordinary measures' and to put him on a breathing machine. Without it there was no hope, though, needless to say—the doctor added—the machine wasn't going to reverse the process of the tumor. . . . And I who had explained to my father the provisions of the living will and got him to sign it, didn't know what to do. . . . How could I take it on myself to decide that my father should be finished with life, life which is ours to know just once. Far from invoking the living will, I was nearly on the verge of ignoring it and saying: "Anything! Anything!"

But Philip backed off: "'Dad, I'm going to have to let you go.' He'd been unconscious for several hours and couldn't hear me, but, shocked, amazed and weeping, I repeated it to him again and then again, until I believed it myself."[16]

Rejecting the respirator takes on the same centrality in Andrew Malcolm's account of the death of his mother. Familiar with hospital routines, having reported on them extensively for the New York Times, Malcolm was still overwhelmed by the sight of his mother in an ICU, suffering through the closing but by no means final stages of metastatic disease. "Medicines and liquids pumped into her immobile arms. Urine dripping out the other end into a plastic bag to be measured and studied to the last milliliter by faceless technicians." In deep distress, he asked the doctor: "What's the outlook?" He was told, "Several months of respiratory therapy, which just might get her lungs functioning enough to maybe get adequate oxygen to the brain to regain consciousness. If nothing else went wrong in the meantime. And then eighteen to twenty-four months down that uncertain road was the lung cancer's likely spread." Malcolm had doubts about going all out. "'Geez, Doc. I'd love to have my mother back. But I wonder about the point to all this.' . . . A deep breath. Oh, God, here we go. A swallowed sob. 'I want to let her go.'" In the end, he had his mother removed from the respirator.[17]

Drawing conclusions about social attitudes from best seller lists is always a treacherous exercise, but the sale of 400,000 copies of Derek Humphry's *Final Exit* did seem to confirm that Americans were persuaded that the primary problem with medicine was that it was doing too much, not too little. The text on how to kill yourself was padded, repetitious, and self-promotional, and the substance did not quite live up to its billing of "self- deliverance." But if additional evidence were needed that doctors and hospitals were overstepping boundaries and forcing their technologies on people, the popularity of *Final Exit* provided it.[18]

The extent to which these various strains combined to give rationing the appearance of acceptability is evidenced in the extraordinarily favorable reception accorded the 1989 proposal by the Oregon legislature to ration health care delivery. Despite numerous and altogether obvious inequities in the plan, many policy analysts, editorial writers, academic commentators, and public officials extolled the effort. Indeed, to judge by the reception accorded Oregon, rationing had now achieved unparalleled approval.

In July of that year, under the leadership of Dr. John Kitzhaber, a former emergency room physician who would later be elected governor, Oregon passed a Basic Health Services Act. It expanded the number of people eligible for Medicaid coverage, but so as not to increase total state expenditures, it cut back the medical benefits recipients could obtain; the retrenchment was so severe that it violated federal minimum standards for Medicaid benefits. According to the act, local citizen forums would discuss the relative importance of different medical services, a state committee would formally rank them in priority (taking into account efficacy, quality of life, and public opinion), an actuarial group would next calculate the cost of each service, and then the legislature would make its annual Medicaid appropriation. The final list of benefits would depend on how far down the list of services the appropriation would go.[19]

Editorial pages celebrated the measure for designing the very kind of rationing the country required. Oregon's effort was a "brave medical experiment"; its legislature was "biting the bullet." It was shrewdly

shifting thousands of dollars from programs that would bring doubtful benefits to a handful of individuals (such as organ transplant procedures) and
allocating them to programs, like prenatal care, certain to promote the
welfare of whole groups. Daniel Callahan considered it a "bold and inte-
grated" plan and Troyen Brennan found it "rational." Since the rankings
had been the subject of public discussion, the consensus was ostensibly
democratically achieved. And because Medicaid benefits were now extended
to an additional 100,000 people, who had heretofore lacked coverage, the
trade-off seemed more than equitable.

Lost in the excitement over Oregon's initiative, however, was the in-
controvertible fact that the restrictions affected only the Medicaid population—the poor bore the exclusive burden of the cutbacks and, in effect,
subsidized the extension of medical coverage to others. To heighten the
inequities, the plan did not affect the entirety of the Medicaid population.
Exempted from it were the elderly, despite the fact that the social and medical services they received amounted to well over half of the Medicaid budget. Social services, Kitzhaber and others responded, were too difficult to
rank; others were convinced that powerful nursing home operators had
effectively lobbied the legislature. Oregon did not even extend its policy to
the state's own medical insurance program for its employees. In effect, everyone was exempted from the rationing exercise—the entire non-Medicaid
population, state employees, the elderly—except for low income women
and their children. Looked at closely, Oregon was less a brave adventure
than a time-honored exercise in penalizing the poor. But rationing seemed
so much the order of the day that so long as the schemes affected someone
else, the reviews were favorable.

Bringing all these developments together, a clever political consultant in
1992, wondering which initiatives would be most welcomed by the elector-
ate in the upcoming campaigns, had ample reason to conclude that a new
and very different series of presumptions now prevailed in the field of health
policy. It might be possible to implement a national health insurance program and, at the same time, contain costs. Why? Because Americans were
apparently discarding their traditional commitments to medical machines,

seeing technology as double-edged, sometimes delivering a miracle, at other times inflicting pain. From this new angle of vision, they might prove willing to make trade-offs, to compromise access to technology in return for other benefits. Rationing might not be an anathema, at least if government took the opportunity to meet other critical needs of the middle classes. After all, who wanted to be tethered to a respirator anyway?

6 | No Limits

A merican health care policy in the early 1990s seemed to be on the verge of a genuine revolution. Even skeptical observers were persuaded that the twin pillars upholding past practices were crumbling and a new departure was imminent. First, as we have seen, Americans were apparently becoming disenchanted with medical technologies, recognizing the need for tough-minded decisions about allocation. But, second, and even more astonishing, the middle classes were becoming acutely dissatisfied with the workings of private health insurance. The marketplace was letting *them* down, not giving them the protections they needed. The concern was not so much about the 40 million uninsured Americans as the fact that the insurance costs of the middle classes were climbing and their coverage was jeopardized if they changed jobs or became unemployed. To a number of political analysts and health economists, these two perspectives, joined together, significantly improved the prospects for national health insurance. Once the middle classes felt the need to make trade-offs, to give up unbounded access to medical machines in return for guaranteed coverage, it might well be possible to provide a health insurance program for all by the year 2000.

The indicators supporting this conclusion were numerous and compelling, ranging from public opinion surveys to election victories. Poll after poll revealed that Americans were prepared to support a basic redesign in health care delivery, not for reasons of altruism but self-interest. A survey commissioned by the Robert Wood Johnson Foundation, a frank advocate for national health insurance, revealed that 85% of Americans favored sweeping changes in health care. Fully one-quarter of them were now concerned about losing their own insurance and almost half believed it might well happen to them in the future. A Cable Network News poll reported that 62% of all Americans believed that health care was a right that the government should guarantee. But in more personal terms, two-thirds reported that in the event of major illness, they would have difficulty in handling the crisis or would not be able to do so at all.[1] There were also widespread complaints about the high cost of medical insurance and a pervasive fear that insurance coverage might be lost.[2] Writing in 1992, Robert Blendon, the highly respected public opinion poll analyst, and his associates concluded that "the synergy of benefit cutbacks and rising health care costs has left middle-class Americans worried about their ability to afford health care services, and terrified that a serious illness would wreak havoc on their household finances." Fully 52% of those making over $50,000 a year feared that health insurance was becoming so expensive that they would not be able to afford it. And 24% of people with private insurance reported that they had "put off medical care" because they could not pay for it (compared to only 13% of people on Medicare). Clearly American health policy had spawned something new, "the worried middle class."[3]

In more general terms, polls indicated that Americans were almost evenly divided in their readiness to substitute government intervention for marketplace forces; but at least among Democrats, independents, and middle income workers, the credo that private insurance could handle the assignment was losing its hold.[4] In effect, the original pact that Blue Cross made with middle-class Americans seemed to be dissolving.

At the same time, disillusionment with private health insurance was affecting one of its most powerful and traditional supporters, major American business corporations. They seemed ready to join a campaign for national health insurance in order to contain their own mounting costs. Automobile manufacturers, for example, insisted that the expense of health care exceeded that of steel in producing a car. They would never compete successfully with the Japanese unless the system was revamped.

Were all these indicators not compelling enough, the issue of national health insurance seemed to have political legs, strong enough, for example, to carry Pennsylvania's Harris Wofford to a Senate seat in a special fall 1991 election. Wofford had been lagging well behind his opponent, the incumbent Richard Thornburgh, until he made health care his issue and began running political advertisement around the slogan, "If criminals have a right to a lawyer, I think working Americans should have the right to a doctor." Wofford went on to defeat Thornburgh by a 55 to 45 margin, and the result was credited to his stance on health care.[5]

However encouraging these findings were for policy initiatives, no one in or out of Washington was naive enough to think such attitudes would unambiguously promote the transformation of an $800 billion industry. Yes, Americans said they would pay additional taxes for health care, but a majority would not go above an additional $10 a month, and most favored taxes on cigarettes and alcohol. Yes, the system did need revamping, but over 70% were satisfied with their own doctor and their own health care situation. When asked if there was a time when they needed medical care but did not get it for economic reasons, only 15% of low income families (under $15,000 a year) and 10% of all respondents said yes. In fact, most Americans did not believe that national health insurance would bring them any personal benefits.

This ambivalence notwithstanding, it was apparent in the fall of 1992 that whatever the results of the presidential contest, health care would be a major item on the political agenda. The country was in for a lesson in the comparative advantages and disadvantages of single-payer systems, "play or pay" insurance mandates for corporations, and managed care and managed competition. Not that citizens were prepared or able to follow the particulars of these proposals; polls continued to find almost universal ignorance about the specifics of each of them. But the concerns seemed acute and with the election of Bill Clinton, a commitment to national health insurance was assured. Public opinion and the stake of a variety of constituencies appeared to give him room to play and win.

Although a comprehensive analysis of why change was not forthcoming must await the personal accounts and the private papers of administration and congressional leaders, a host of articles and books have already begun the task of analysis, and some archival materials, including 268 boxes of the Clinton Health Care Reform Task Force, are already available. The framers of the Health Security Act believed that they had the right strategies for designing a political program consistent with prevailing social values, that American attitudes could be made compatible with national health insurance. They proved to be wrong, very wrong, fundamentally misreading the perspectives that Americans bring to health care.

It is political scientists who to date have had the most to say about the causes for the Clinton failure, and their interpretations, as might be expected, follow the schools of thought that they represent within the discipline. The "institutionalists" put the blame squarely on the organization of government, finding it of no surprise that a system designed to build in gridlock cannot effect so fundamental a change. As Sven Steinmo and Jon Watts phrase it: "This fragmentation of political power . . . offered the opponents of reform many opportunities to attack Clinton's plan. This institutional bias, not flaws in the plan or the political strategy . . . once again killed . . . comprehensive NHI in America."[6] Others, including Robert Blendon, fault the public for sending altogether confusing messages to Washington. Because it never mastered the details of the various proposals, it was not capable of making its preferences known and in this way "contributed to Congressional dead-lock."[7] Still others focus on the combined effects of a broad distrust of government and the need for a balanced budget. As Theda Skocpol argues, the Clinton plan had to be "designed to get around and through the anti-government and fiscal legacies of the Reagan era," and in the process it, seem-ingly inevitably, raised cries of governmental tyranny and spendthriftiness.[8] Finally, skilled journalists, like Haynes Johnson and David Broder, have reviewed the day-to-day political events, identifying many gross errors in tactics. The list is almost endless. Giving so much prominence to Hillary Clinton restricted the president's maneuverability, and placing an outsider to Washington, Ira Magaziner, in charge of policy design guaranteed po-litical trouble. Then just when the president was getting ready to focus on health care he had to devote his attention to a crisis in Somalia and an all-out battle to pass NAFTA. In brief, the cause of the failure rests somewhere between bad judgment and bad luck.

For all the persuasiveness of these explanations, they tend to empha-size process more than substance, to give more room to the play of politics and less to the actual content of the plan, and the way that it was presented to and understood by the general public. In fact, one root cause for the debacle, albeit not the only one, was a fundamental misreading of what the public wanted and expected from medicine. Proponents of the Health Se-curity Act tried desperately to connect it to the past, most assiduously to the implementation of the Social Security Act and Medicare. They believed that in light of the contemporary reactions to negative aspects of medical tech-nologies and the anxieties about private health insurance, they could cir-cumvent fears of government involvement and a possible reduction in ac-cess to medicine. But in fact, as we shall see, past values had not lost their relevance or their potency.

The Clinton program, while by no means simple, was hardly as Rube Goldberg–like as critics suggested. The dilemma it sought to resolve was daunting: how to reduce health care costs and maintain access to services for middle-class Americans and at the same time bring an additional 40 million Americans into the system, and to accomplish all this without increasing federal government expenditures and sparking a reaction against big and intrusive government. Were access and cost containment not so intertwined, the solution to national health insurance would have been simple. It only required dropping the age requirement for Medicare and allowing anyone who wanted to enroll to do so. The problem, however, was that Medicare expenditures, even after the introduction of some cost-limiting procedures in the 1980s (such as prospective payments to hospitals based on diagnostic related groupings), were still substantial. One estimate, made for Robert Rubin, then in charge of the president's National Economic Council, put the Medicare percentage increase at 14.4% annually between 1970 and 1990. Were its rolls to swell, costs would be astronomical, no less than $60 billion a year, maybe even double that.[9]

Hence the Clinton team was convinced it had no choice but to reconstruct the health delivery system almost from scratch. Expenditures were already out of control and expanding access might be the straw that broke the proverbial budget back. So if the rallying cry in the election campaign was "The Economy Stupid," in the health care reform arena it was, "Cost Containment." As one White House advisor recounted to Ira Magaziner, he had tried at the end of a meeting to explain to Hillary Clinton one complicated facet of the proposed plan. But before he could finish a sentence, she said, "But we need cost containment," and darted off.[10]

The eventual Clinton solution was to create a network of public regional alliances which would oversee private competition among health plans. Regulation by the alliances would maintain quality and guarantee a level playing field (no plan would be allowed to cream the healthiest subscribers or offer too meager a package of benefits). Competition among the plans would drive down costs. The glory and the drawback of the scheme was its frankly hybrid character, its mix of free enterprise and government oversight. To left-minded critics, it gave too much responsibility to the private sector, allowing profit-oriented companies (who were likely to organize and control the health plans) to continue their dominant role in health care. To politically right-minded critics, the alliances represented enormous state and federal regulation. An $800 billion industry would have to answer to regional alliances which, in turn, would have to answer to Washington.

These objections notwithstanding, the Clinton team thought its design represented a viable compromise, capturing the best of the private and the public sectors. Walter Zelman, former executive director of California Common Cause and the member of the White House staff most instrumental in fashioning this part of the plan, was convinced that the plan's composite character was its greatest strength. "Managed competition," he explained time and again to doubters inside and outside the administration, "is, in fact, a compromise between competitive and regulatory reform approaches. It focuses on market forces but insists those forces be directed . . . to serve consumer, not insurer, ends." It adopted the tactics "generally associated with conservatives (competition) to achieve the ends generally associated with liberals (universal access)."[11] "We can, in fact, appeal to both liberals and conservatives, with different aspects of our package, and not be talking out of both sides of our mouth. . . . We have something that, I think, we can really be proud of—a true political breakthrough, and new possibility of achieving the kind of consensus we've never gotten to before."[12]

Although the administration believed that competition among health care plans would control expenditures, it was not prepared to trust completely to marketplace forces. The prospect of costs escalating wildly was simply too scary; moreover, the proposed legislation did have to win the support of the watchdog Congressional Budget Office (CBO). Accordingly, the plan included a budget cap on total expenditures. By 1996, with the program phased in and the percentage of GNP devoted to health allowed to rise to 16.9%, premiums for health insurance, the pot from which expenditures would come, would not be allowed to exceed the rate of inflation.

Precisely how the cap would work was subject to a variety of explanations but all of them raised the same question: Was this price control under another name? In fact, the Task Force analyzed fully and then rejected applying price controls to health care. Were the administration to impose them in this one sector but no other, resources and personnel would flee health care and go elsewhere. Why work for a hospital with a wage that was frozen if one could take a job in another sector and receive regular wage hikes? Why should a corporation make machines for physicians to use (under a price cap) if it could make machines for others to use (without a price cap)? And although a freeze could regulate the prices charged, how would it go about limiting volume? Tell physicians that they can only charge so much for an office visit, and, as was learned from the Nixon price freeze experience, physicians would then see more patients in the course of a day and have more patients make return visits. If economics is a dismal science, health care explains why.[13]

Even more ominously, was the provision of a cap in the health care plan rationing under another name? In fact, one of the major reasons that the Clinton plan failed was its inability to handle this question satisfactorily. The plan followed a strategy of reticence and restraint, which bred an extraordinary amount of suspicion and hostility. It was over the issue of budget caps that opponents of the Clinton plan went to the public and succeeded in casting doubt on the integrity of the entire effort. Over budget caps the middle classes deserted Clinton and thus, once again, national health insurance was defeated.

Budget caps were the part of the health plan package that the Clinton forces were least eager to talk about. From their perspective, it was the backup, fail-safe option that had to be invoked to make the whole package financially credible. If all the pieces worked well, no one would bump up against them. Caps could not be eliminated from the program—the CBO insisted that it would never sanction a program that did not have enforceable limits. (And the CBO, let it be said, was delighted with the caps as designed; "We looked for big loopholes," remarked one of its economists, "and we couldn't find any.")[14] But the administration was not willing to emphasize this element. The glory of the program lay in relieving the anxieties of middle-class families about retaining and paying for their health insurance policies and bringing the benefits of national coverage to needy families. The caps were a means to this end, not an end in themselves.

When forced to elaborate on how the caps would work in practice, the Clinton officials responded as tersely as possible. In the public policy literature, they did offer some explanations, all of which minimized the pain and discomfort that caps might possibly cause. Paul Starr, a close adviser to the White House during the development of the plan, offered several reasons not to be alarmed about them. For one, a plan that allowed 16.9% of GNP to go to health care provided sufficient leeway for Americans to get all the medicine that was good for them. For another, American medicine had a well-deserved reputation for delivering too much, not only in terms of forcing people onto respirators, but performing an excessive number of procedures. The caps would help instill "a high quality but conservative practice style—conservative in the sense of conserving resources by proceeding with treatment only when clearly effective."[15] And to make certain that no one mistook "conservative" for niggardliness, Starr insisted that caps would promote a long overdue change both in the economics and in the psychology of health care decision making. Budget considerations would encourage "managers and physicians to concentrate instead on using resources well. Instead of promoting an aggressive style and an emphasis on high cost procedures, global caps encourage less resource-intense practices that enable providers to manage under constraint. . . . America's traditional payment system has nurtured therapeutic activism ('when in doubt, take it out'); budget limits nurture therapeutic skepticism ('let's wait and see how this develops')." Thus individuals did not have to be worried about the implications of this new orientation for the quality of the health care they received. "Given the abundant evidence of excessive surgery, overprescribing, and unnecessary hospitalization," declared Starr, "a strong dose of skepticism seems overdue."[16] It was as if the invisible hand of Adam Smith had returned to right the balance in medicine. Under budget caps the pendulum would swing back from excess to just the proper midpoint on the arc.

Moreover, Starr insisted, the caps were not threatening because American medicine had extravagant waste built into it. Impose a fixed limit along with managed competition, and the money saved would obviate any need to limit effective interventions. Were all these points not persuasive enough, Starr contended that even were the Clinton plan scuttled, caps would eventually have to be invoked because health costs would continue to mount. And, he hastened to explain, caps were not an exercise in rationing, if what one meant by rationing was an Oregon-type plan that set down rules in advance about which medical procedures could or could not be performed. He did concede, without elaboration, that "Global budgeting may require tough choices." But he never defined explicitly what these choices might be, preferring instead to observe that they would be made not by state administrators (as enemies of big government might fear) but by "the changing judgments and negotiations of health plan managers, doctors, and patients. . . . This approach avoids the rigidity of detailed official rules that are likely to become outdated as new scientific discoveries emerge."[17] In all, setting limits would only improve practices. Caps were good for both patient and society.

Walter Zelman was no less confident that the budget caps were a "backstop cost containment mechanism" that should please tax-conscious citizens and corporations alike. "It is neither economically appropriate nor politically viable," Zelman contended, "to require that families or businesses make a substantial contribution for health care and then have to face premium increases of 15% or more, as they have so often in recent years." But he, too, conceded, again without being specific, that budget caps might prove troublesome. "No one should anticipate that such a backstop cost control mechanism will be without controversy. But unless we are prepared to tell employers, individuals, and the government itself that their liability is unlimited . . . such a backstop is even more necessary than it is controversial."[18]

The Question and Answer materials prepared in the White House to guide the administration's public presentation of the health care plan warily obfuscated the issue of caps and the inexorably related issue of rationing.[19] The section for "Consumers and Health Care" laid out a script that went:

Q: Will my care be limited in any way?
A: No. . . . Health plans competing on the basis of service and quality to attract and retain patients . . . will have every incentive to provide necessary care on a timely basis.

For the "Physicians and Health Care" section, the proposed dialogue went:

Q: As a doctor, I'm concerned that budgeting will lead to rationed care and poor quality medicine. How can we be sure that won't happen?
A: . . . Throughout the United States, innovative corporations, group practices, and health care institutions have proven that cost-effective care does not reduce quality; in fact, it increases it.

And then under the "Controlling Costs" section:

Q: Will the national budget cause my health care to be rationed?

A: . . . The truth is that we spend more than we should on health care right now. . . . Billions of dollars are wasted in administrative expenses and unnecessary tests and procedures. The national health care budget will impose some discipline on our health care spending and insure that appropriate care is provided as efficiently as possible.

Nowhere do these materials confront directly the possibility that imposing a cap would impose a constraint on services and compel physicians or the health care plans or the regional alliances to exercise choice among effective interventions, that is, to ration care. Perhaps eliminating waste and letting expenditures climb to 16.9% of the budget would obviate the need. But there was a potential conflict that the White House preferred not to acknowledge. Better to keep the matter under wraps.

The one internal demurral to this proposition came from the Ethics section of the Task Force. Most of this group's work went into formulating the "Ethical Foundations of the New Health Care System," including "The Fundamental Moral Importance of Health Care" (health care *is* different), the need for "Wise Allocation" (health care is not Americans' only value), and for "Generational Solidarity" (the needs of the young should not be in conflict with the needs of the elderly).[20] But in April 1993, the group sent Ira Magaziner a "Personal Memorandum" on "Wise Resource Allocation and Limits to Health Services." Noting that "Because this is a sensitive political issue, we raise it in this memo rather than in the more public tollgate [joint Task Force meetings] context."[21]

The memo immediately went to the core of the issue. The presumption among the architects of health care reform appeared to be that "cost savings from the new reforms will be sufficient to make unnecessary any significant limitations on beneficial care. . . . We believe that this assumption is false. . . . Many of us believe that the issue of limitations on care should be addressed both for ethical and political reasons." The text went on to argue that however much waste was eliminated, advances in technology will drive up costs and make hard choices necessary. Moreover, "we do not now and would not want in the future to provide every beneficial health care service to all, regardless how small its benefit and how great its costs." Indeed, the memo warned, not to address this issue would be to play into the hands of opponents of reform. "The plan's critics will undoubtedly raise the issue of limitations on care—and it will be given the inflammatory label of rationing and cannot be swept under the rug in the political debate." Finally, "limitations on care is one of the fundamental ethical issues in healthcare reform," and, as such, warrants exploration. As against those who defended covert decision making on the grounds that the "social costs of an open process are too high," this group insisted that fairness would be achieved only through public discussion. However, its exhortation had no impact. Whether for reasons of social costs or political costs, the Clinton administration chose not to confront the issue.

Not only the administration but some health policy analysts, like Jack Hadley and Stephen Zuckerman, were convinced that concerns about the impact of the caps, notably "the specter of sick patients being unable to receive care," represented "fear-mongering." The American system was so inflated—they estimated that waste of resources in hospitals amounted to $50–$70 billion—that the prospect of a cap would provide incentives to become cost-effective without reducing the quality of patient care.[22] Apparently, the advantage of inheriting so bloated a system was that change could come with a minimum of undesirable side effects.

The administration's desire to duck the issue of caps or, when pushed, to contend that eliminating waste and inefficiency obviated all problems, was evident to a number of shrewd policy analysts, and several of them commented on it. Mark Pauly, professor of economics and business at the University of Pennsylvania, observed that everyone believed that the "achievement of the goals of universal coverage and cost containment requires some wrenching trade-offs." But the rhetoric surrounding the plan, he observed, "has emphasized neither painful consequences nor trade-offs." Pauly wondered, as did many others: "What happened to the tough choices?"[23]

Pauly was not alone in his skepticism. Daniel Mendelson, another policy analyst, estimated that waste represented only 1.5% of the nation's health care bill. Hence, "a few years down the line, you first start to see what we call silent rationing, where the patients don't even know that they're not receiving the beneficial care that they need. Further down the line, I think it would become very clear that we were denying patients some of the latest technology in order to save money."[24]

Henry Aaron, one of the most sophisticated health economists, also took note of the silence around budget caps, explaining it in terms of the political maxim of "Never be seen to do direct harm." Since health reform unavoidably "must do some harm," either by raising taxes to pay the costs or by limiting the incomes of health care providers, politicians did not want to address yet another problem. Aaron himself had no quarrel with budget caps. "President Clinton's repeated insistence that national spending limits are essential for the sustained control of growth of spending is correct." No other mechanism will provide incentives to increase efficiency and cut costs. But, he accurately predicted, the cap issue would prove explosive. No matter how assiduously the administration tried to obfuscate the fact, "large reductions in the growth of health care spending eventually must force the denial of some beneficial care to some people." Sooner or later, budget caps were going to mean that a patient would be unable to receive an intervention that would do him good. "Despite the palpable truth of this assertion," concluded Aaron, "it is more effective in emptying a room of elected officials than shouting 'fire.'" In the end, "the choices that rationing will impose are ethically and politically distressing," and render it likely that despite all efforts to be "fuzzing this truth," Clinton's national health budget and budget caps "will fail to win majority support."[25]

Still other commentators agonized over how best to present ideas on rationing to the public, but nothing that was said led the Clinton administration to address the issue forthrightly. Victor Fuchs, an economist especially sensitive to social determinants of policy, was deeply concerned about the divergences created by a health reform system charged both to cap expenditures and to meet the potential demand for more services. "What kind of health policy," he wondered, "would keep the insured elderly from demanding and receiving all the care that might do them some good without regard to cost?" He did concede that the current "discussion and debate over the right to death with dignity," with its commitment to the patient's right to refuse treatment and obtain physician assistance in ending life might brake expenditures. But he worried that "as financial and ethical pressures mount, we probably will see the right to death with dignity transformed into an expectation and eventually into an obligation." Perhaps the elderly would be willing to trade high-tech (and expensive) medical services that added a short period to their lives for low-tech (and inexpensive) services, like housing, transportation, and assistance with shopping, that improved the quality of their lives. But to Fuchs, Americans were on the horns of a dilemma: no one could be confident that the low-tech choice would be popular and yet, the system would not be able to cope with "the potentially unlimited demand for health care by the elderly."[26] Thus Fuchs, like Aaron, was deeply pessimistic about the prospects for change.

Not only economists but an occasional bioethicist complained about the administration's not coming out front on the issue of rationing. Writing in the *Christian Century*, Allen Verhey, director of the Institute of Religion at the Texas Medical Center in Houston, argued that the "optimism of the Clinton plan is self-deceptive, and its description of necessary choices . . . as simply 'medical' choices is potentially self-destructive. . . . It nurtures little public awareness of the necessity and hard reality of these choices." He perceptively noted that "the story of the frontier does not train those who tell it to be content with limits," and that "President Clinton drew no narrative lines from the story he plotted to our discontent with limits . . . or to our suspicion of nature and our confidence in technology." In sum, "we Americans [must] revise our larger story to fix the health care problem."[27]

However standard and predictable the reticence of the Clinton administration about caps, its strategy turned out to be fatal to the cause of national health insurance. What the silence did, however unintended, was to hand the issue of rationing over to the opposition. It was around caps and imposed scarcity that the foes of national health insurance captured public attention—and helped to drive down public support for the measure. In April 1993, 71% of the public supported the plan; in April 1994, the percentage dropped to 43, with notable losses among the middle classes.[28] In large measure, they deserted the Clinton plan over the prospect of rationing.

Perhaps it was inevitable that caps would have sooner or later turned the middle classes against the program. No matter what Clinton said, rationing would have cast its shadow over reform. Survey research reported that "the public does not see the need to make major sacrifices themselves in order to bring the system under control." Doctors, lawyers, hospitals, and insurance companies ought to bear the burden of containment, not patients.

The problem with American health care was the greed of the providers, not the demands of the patients. "By margins of roughly three-to-one," reported one analysis, "Americans oppose rationing health care (76% to 21%) [or] rationing care for the elderly (73% to 24%)."[29]

But the tactic of ducking the issue or squeezing it in as a throw-away line between arguments about eliminating waste and overtreatment had an ominous side effect. It provided the opposition with the occasion to explore the potential mischief that rationing would create and to present its arguments as though it had uncovered the dirty little secret of the Clinton administration. There was an exposé quality to the criticisms of rationing; the plan was condemned on its merits and for trying to disguise its true consequences. Critics were able to assert that what was at stake in the debate was not only rationing but trust, a formulation that was particularly effective against a president who never managed to inspire trust. Thus to bring the two messages together, how could a government that would try to delude the American public about such a scheme ever be allowed to make life–death decisions about individual health care?[30]

The most striking finding that emerges from an examination of the health care debate as it took place in the nation's newspapers and popular magazines is the extent to which rationing became the club with which to beat on the Clinton health initiative. The dreaded L word that was used so effectively in the 1980s to tar the Democratic Party as free-spenders with middle class money was succeeded by the "dreaded R word," to tar the Health Security Act as a death-dealing plan.[31] Rationing was not just something that would be done to the poor—it would now be done to you, the middle classes. It was one thing to decide that one's parent or child should not remain comatose on a respirator, quite another to have freedom of choice about the use of medical technology taken away by the government.

An extraordinarily diverse coalition spread the message that national health care meant rationing of all medicine for all Americans. It came from members of the political right, the religious right, and disabilities organizations, along with insurance companies, business associations, individual corporations, taxpayer groups, and health care providers. Preachers, senators, representatives, and would-be officeholders each found in rationing the Achilles' heel of the program. Not that it served as the sole grounds for objection. There was no shortage of claims that national health insurance would bankrupt the treasury, deny Americans the freedom to choose their doctors, impose unconscionable delays on patients, and ruin the professional practice of medicine. There was plenty of language to the effect that the Clinton plan "interposes a massive government bureaucracy between individuals and their physicians," and makes doctors into the "agents of the state." But all these more general points were made immediate and personal through the descriptions of the gross abuses that rationing would inevitably bring.

One might have anticipated that the more conservative groups in American society would embrace the idea of budget caps, seeing it as an effective method for curbing expenditure. And although the government did set the cap, it did not itself decide exactly which expenditures would be limited. But that was not the stance that the political right adopted. Determined to defeat the plan for any one of a number of reasons, it shrewdly manipulated the issue of caps so as to galvanize the opposition of the middle classes. Ultimately, it was able to convince the public that the Clinton plan would cost them more money and deliver them less medicine. Whatever degree of discomfort the middle classes experienced because of the cost and restrictions of private health insurance, they were still better off than having the government tell them what treatments they could or could not receive from their doctors.

The religious right was particularly energetic in using rationing to make its case. Unhappy at the prospect of government intervention in general but furious at a program that threatened to use federal funds for abortion, its members were indefatigable in their efforts to defeat the bill. Pat Robertson's Christian Coalition, for example, announced it was spending $1.4 million to lobby against the plan through radio and newspaper advertisements, direct mail, and telephone calls; it was also sending 30 million postcards criticizing the plan to the members of 60,000 churches. Indeed, the Christian Coalition wanted to use the issue of rationing to widen its circle of supporters, contending that officials who were on the record as being in favor of killing fetuses would next be killing the elderly. A government that was ready to end life in its earliest stages would be a government ready to end life in its later stages. As Joseph Messner, head of the Greater Cleveland Right to Life insisted, the Health Security Act should be called the Health Rationing Act, "because the proposed law's cost controls could, over time, give bureaucrats decisive power over a patient's care. That could mean a given patient's age, physical condition, or nebulous 'quality of life' might not entitle him or her to full-blown medical treatment." Or as C. Ben Mitchell, speaking for the Southern Baptist Convention, declared: "End-of-life decisions should not be predicated strictly upon economic restraints or government protocols. Neither should health care be rationed or restricted based upon the age, quality of life, or disability of the patient."[32]

Conservative Republicans eagerly took up the cause and tried to make political capital of it. New Jersey Congresswoman Marge Roukema introduced an amendment to the health care bill entitled: "To Preserve Patient/ Doctor Choice and to Eliminate Rationing." In the Senate, Republican Don Nickles, from Oklahoma, introduced the Consumer Choice Health Security Act, which explicitly ruled out rationing medical care.[33]

Health care providers felt especially comfortable in framing their opposition to the plan in terms of rationing. Duane Dauner, president of the California Association of Hospitals and Health Systems, denounced it as "a one-way ticket to rationing of health care. Doctors, nurses, care providers and — most important — patients would be forced to take their marching orders from a state health czar and an army of bureaucrats."[34] Dr. George Fisher, writing in *USA Today* centered his opposition on the fact that one way or another, the Clinton initiative meant less medicine, either by direct rationing or, indirectly, by reducing the number of specialists. Patients would not be able to get necessary but expensive treatments for treating incontinence, for example, if there were no urologists around. (And citing the example of incontinence was not a random choice.)[35] These same cautions were voiced by the president of St. Joseph's Hospital in Phoenix: "No one wants to talk about rationing, but that's where we're headed." Lee Peterson, the chief executive of the Sun Health Corporation, even cited William Knaus's Apache ICU program to buttress his vision for the future with rationing. "What we may see happen," he predicted, "is the third-party payer will say, 'If the chance of survival is below 5 percent, we're not going to pay for whatever treatment you are considering.'"[36]

To these voices were added the advocates for the disabilities community. Paul Malek, representing one such Denver-based group, maintained
that in adopting the Clinton plan Americans would be following a
"Dr. Kevorkian" approach to health care. "Though we don't like to openly
discuss it, we are coming to an era [in which] we may not want to spend
scarce resources on people with disabilities."[37] This same theme was reiterated by the journalist Nat Hentoff, who some years before had expressed
outrage when parents of a defective newborn in New York were able to
convince a neonatologist not to pursue heroic treatment. "To achieve universal health care," Hentoff contended, "it would seem the government can
condemn people to death for having an inappropriate 'quality of life.'"[38]
Organizations of the elderly also worried deeply about this possibility. The
Denver-based Senior's Coalition told its members, and others, that the
Clinton plan was designed to "put them at the end of the rationing list." It
would be the elderly who would be the target of the cutbacks.[39]

Ad hoc as well as more established conservative organizations spread
these ideas still deeper through the public. Citizens for Choice in Health
Care, based in St. Paul, Minnesota, invoked decision making around the
respirator to make its point: "True compassionate health care will find itself in need of resuscitation without an available life support unit. . . . Later
we will wonder how we let the 2,000-year-old Hippocratic oath of patient as
primary be rendered impractical against the concept of a global budget."
The Citizens Against Rationing Health, allied with the American Conservative Union and the Heritage Foundation, asserted that the Clinton cure
for rationing was far worse than the disease.[40]

These comments took on added import because they effectively presented rationing as the scandal uncovered. No one better captured the tone
of exposing a hidden truth than Elizabeth McCaughey, writing in the *New
Republic*.[41] A novice in the health care field with no special expertise, and
affiliated with a conservative think tank in Manhattan, McCaughey successfully presented her attack as ferreting out a duplicitous scheme. She was
frequently quoted in the press (especially by those opposed to the plan), was
the object of a special rebuttal from the White House (which only gave her
more publicity), and, in the process, helped make national health insurance
synonymous with rationing and government distrust. (For her efforts, she

became George Pataki's running mate in the 1994 New York gubernatorial election and won the election for lieutenant governor.)

McCaughey argued that Americans did not know what the Health Security Act contained, not because it was over 1300 pages long but because "you haven't been given a straight story about the Clinton health bill." And what that straight story will tell you—implicitly the middle-class "you"—is that costs will grow and services shrink. Because of the caps, she declared, "The health care you get will be limited." To provide vignettes of precisely what this would mean, she drew on every horror story ever perpetuated about an HMO that restricted treatment. Those with backaches will not be able to get surgery for disc removal; patients will have to wait for tests and treatment until a nurse and a clerk at an 800 number approve the doctor's decision. All physicians will have to follow "cook-book medicine." Underscoring the traditional values that Americans have brought to health care, McCaughey went on to argue that under the Clinton plan, "You'll get more primary care medicine than high-tech medicine, and that's not good news." No bypass surgery, no angioplasty, no specialists. Explaining the purported "unwritten rationing rules," she observed that the government was hiding its intentions by promising to deliver all medical care that was "necessary" and "appropriate." But, she noted, it would be a presidentially appointed management board that would define what these terms meant, not the doctor or the patient. And under this arrangement, she predicted, more attention would be paid to cost-saving than to individual well-being. "When a kidney transplant is needed, will the patient's age matter, as it does in Great Britain, where older patients are routinely denied high-tech treatment?" Are we all to come under "an Oregon like system, where advanced cases of cancer go untreated?"

Because of the administration's silence on the rationing issue, McCaughey's tactics were effective enough to withstand the challenges from numerous critics who pointed out specific errors in her presentation. Indeed, to make matters worse, the Health Security Act could not at this point set out elaborate definitions of what was or was not to be considered medically necessary and appropriate—it was leaving that task to the deliberations of a newly created board. But the result of that decision was to make the bill vulnerable to just the sort of attack McCaughey launched. Imagine your favorite medical intervention—and imagine it left off the roster of allowable procedures.

The Health Security Act also provoked a series of attacks from the Health Insurance Association of America, the "Harry and Louise" series of political advertisements. In retrospect, their prominence may owe less to a blanketing of the market—they were shown mostly in New York, Washington, D.C., and on CNN, in an effort to influence the press—than to the attention that the Clinton administration and its supporters devoted to denouncing them. The intensity of their reactions reflected the fact that Harry and Louise were the quintessential middle-class, really upper-middle-class, couple, the very core of the supporters that the administration wanted to attract, and the message they delivered was effectively aimed to arouse opposition to the plan.

Harry and Louise, in the thirteen episodes in which they appeared, lived in a gracious home and drove an expensive car. They were raising two children while both held down good jobs—Louise has several conversations with her black administrative aide in the office. Even more important, both carried private insurance (there are references to "plans like ours"); indeed, Louise's company offered very good benefits—which, she declared, ought not to be taxed as the Clinton plan proposed. Harry and Louise were not against a national health insurance program (this point was made repeatedly), but they were opposed to the Clinton plan. Several of the episodes show Louise reading the published version of the plan (in her well-appointed living room), and at the end of almost each segment, she promises to write to tell her congressman that there has "got to be a better way." She is confident "Congress can fix that." The tone is one of reasoned consideration, political engagement, and active concern. These are good people who have everyone's interest at heart. Some critics notwithstanding, the frames are the opposite end of the spectrum from the Willy Horton ads.[42]

What troubled Harry and Louise most? First, the potential intrusiveness of the government bureaucrats. "They choose, we lose," was one refrain; do we really want to create a "billion dollar bureaucracy?" another. The plan represents "just too much government." Second, and still more prominently, the prospect of rationing of medical care. "What if our health care plan runs out of money?" Louise asks in several episodes. To her, the plan is "rationing, the way I read it," with long waiting lines and "some services not even available." Louise wanted private insurance (as per the sponsors of the series) and "no spending limits." The Clinton readiness to place "limits on health care spending" becomes "some kind of rationing." "Limits on spending just logically has to mean limits on services." In sum, Harry and Louise posed the very question that the Clinton plan most wanted to avoid. They were defining the plan in just the way the Clintons feared, that is, one that gave to the poor by taking from the middle class. It was a design that doesn't help "us," but "them." We are better off with what we have than with what the bureaucrats won't give us.*

A number of attorneys who analyzed the plan also wrote about rationing with the air of exposing an alarming secret. Trained to devise worst case scenarios, they had a field day with the many questions that the Clinton plan could not resolve in advance, even to the point of debating the legal liabilities of HMOs that followed rationing guidelines.[43] To be sure, the administration promised that cutting waste would obviate the need to invoke caps. But cutting waste, like supply side economics in the Reagan administration, seemed nothing more than wishful thinking. As one attorney observed: "The greatest fear is that reform will not achieve its promises, and that it will eventually be forced by financial pressures to ration medically necessary care. . . . There is no effective means for restraining the rise in health care costs except by denying access. . . . The tradeoff for universal health care coverage is a system of lesser capabilities that substitutes explicit rationing for today's hodgepodge of cost control. . . . The allocation of limited health care resources is an issue that will not go away and needs to be addressed as part of the debate on health care reform."[44]

Responses came back. Some columnists labeled the attack on rationing a classic "red herring" tactic. But the arguments that followed were often variations on the theme that no one should be disturbed by rationing be-

---

*The Clintons' best rejoinder to the advertisements actually did not confront the message. With Bill and Hillary playing Harry and Louise in fine comic style, Hillary faulted the health care plan because people would still die under it. It was cleverly done, but implicitly, and perhaps not even consciously, suggested that more medicine was not a solution to our mortality. Whether the middle class is ready to accept this message remains uncertain.

cause we did it already. That rejoinder, of course, missed the point insofar as the middle classes were concerned, for the rationing that already existed penalized the poor, not them. The Clinton plan would include them—and hence the anxiety.

A few supporters of the health plan attempted to tell the story straight, but they were lone voices, did not speak for the administration, and were remarkably unskilled at making the case for rationing in a palatable fashion. Thus C. Everett Koop, the former Surgeon-General, addressed the question of how much health care each American would receive under the new system and was ready to invoke "the word no one wants to use—rationing." "We've got to find a way," he insisted, "to communicate to all Americans that we cannot have every procedure or every test every time we want and still control health care spending." In a tone certain to offend the middle classes, he concluded that to enact new initiatives required curbing "not just greed among some insurers, providers and special interests, but also greed among patients."[45]

Rhetoric aside, why were the middle classes so resistant to the prospect of limiting medicine? Why was it that the trends that seemed to be emerging in the early 1990s did not translate into a readiness to run the risks of trade-offs? Part of the reason is specific to the Clinton administration. As poll after poll has demonstrated, this president, elected by a minority of the voting public, did not inspire trust. He was not a man easily deferred to about life–death choices.

But more important still was a basic misreading of what precisely the early 1990s' attitudes had represented. The Clinton supporters were misled by the favorable press and professional reactions to a rationing scheme like Oregon's and to the literature that tried to fashion ethically acceptable rationing standards. They accepted too quickly the notion that the respirator represented all that was wrong in American medicine and so long as one did not draw too much attention to it, the middle classes might be prepared to compromise access in return for the security of national health insurance. Had the iron lung and the dialysis machine been more prominent in their analysis, had they reckoned more fully with the American Way in health care, they would have better appreciated all that is special to the middle classes about high-tech medicine.

Would a different posture toward rationing and caps have made a difference? Would a frank appeal for trade-offs have maintained the support of the middle classes for the plan? At the least, candor might have prevented or counterbalanced the devastating critiques that opponents offered in terms of rationing. Ignoring the issue only served to make it more sinister. To be sure, the administration might not have been able to persuade the middle classes to take the step. American values about access to medical machines and middle-class sensibilities about securing their own interests fully before worrying about the position of the less privileged remained very powerful. But when confronting such a tradition, silence and obfuscation are almost certain to fail, indeed, to breed suspicion and even paranoia. In this sense, the Clinton defeat makes it that much more difficult in the future to win the sympathy of the middle classes for national health insurance.

Epilogue

In the three years that have followed the defeat of the Clinton health care initiative, the design of the American health care system has been transformed, not because of anything that has been accomplished in Washington, but because of the workings of the marketplace. The resounding losses that Democratic congressional candidates suffered in the election of 1994, and the dramatic but short-lived ascendancy of Gingrich Republicanism immediately thereafter, guaranteed that health care would be relegated to the margins of the national political agenda. But at the same time, the pressures that had forced the administration to redesign medical services continued to operate with undiminished intensity. If anything they accelerated, because everyone recognized that political solutions were not forthcoming. Thus the major stakeholders in health care, particularly the corporations that have to pay employee medical benefits, realized that they would have to come up with their own solutions to the financial problems posed by providing unlimited access to high technology medicine. Once it became clear that Washington would have nothing to offer, they pursued and implemented their own solutions.

The result has been an accelerated shift from fee-for-service medicine to managed care, a shift that has implications for almost every aspect of health care delivery. In the mid-1980s, 95% of workers who enjoyed employer-sponsored health benefits were under a fee-for-service arrangement. Now only 50% are. The rest are enrolled in managed care, usually as members of health maintenance organizations. So, too, some 20 million Medicare recipients are currently receiving their medical services through managed care, and no less than 35 states have enrolled some or all of their Medicaid recipients in these organizations as well.[1]

The differences between the two arrangements are fundamental. Under fee-for-service, patients select their own physicians and together they make choices about treatment; they do face some external constraints, since third party payers, such as Blue Cross, impose payment schedules and will not cover all services (like cosmetic surgery or experimental treatments). But as a rough rule, fee-for-service gives patients and physicians considerable latitude in making their decisions. Under managed care, patients must select their physicians from a roster of participants in their particular plan, and treatment choices must conform to the practice standards of the managed care organization and be congruous with the financial incentives or penalties it places on physicians. (As health care analysts properly note, "physician practice is what is 'managed' in managed care.")[2] The details vary from HMO to HMO, but managed care alters underlying incentives. In fee-for-service, the inducement has been to treat more. In managed care, it is to treat less. Indeed, in for-profit managed care, which is fast becoming the dominant form of organization, the inducements to treat less are likely to be even more intense.

Managed care, in the guise of managed competition, was integral to Clinton's health care initiative, and the very concerns that opponents voiced about denials of treatment and rationing in the proposed act are equally applicable to the existing programs. The major difference, of course, is in the locus of responsibility. In the Clinton plan, the government would have been the ultimate regulating force. In managed care as it is now developing, it is the marketplace. Indeed, political observers have commented that Clinton was lucky to have his plan defeated—otherwise it would be his regulators, not the HMO executives, that would be making the hard choices, denying payments, and bearing the brunt of intense resentment.

In light of traditional American attitudes and practices, the outstanding issue is how managed care will be reconciled with middle-class insistence on enjoying practically unfettered access to medical technologies. Heretofore, private insurance and unlimited supply went hand in hand, and when private insurance lagged in its ability to deliver access, the federal government stepped in, as exemplified by Medicare and the end-stage renal disease program. But the formula no longer holds. For the first time,

Americans are confronting a system in which private insurance and restricted access go hand in hand, a marketplace that does what was heretofore unthinkable for the middle classes—one that rations medical technology. Clinton learned, as the political scientist Lawrence Jacobs remarked, that it was "politically treacherous to attempt to restructure the supply of high-technology care," even as it was "financially ruinous to open access to an unrestrained supply of ever-developing medical technology."[3] But managed care is now being forced to confront this identical dilemma. How will it prevent a revolt among consumers even as it attempts to limit supply?

To judge by the tales of managed care recounted in the media, the declarations of medical societies, the investigative articles by medical researchers, along with the agitation of particular patients and the enactments of state legislatures, it will not be easy. All of them have focused attention on the degree to which managed care currently restricts, or will restrict, access to high technology medicine. There is general agreement that the structural arrangements to do so are in place—which is why the prospect of rationing provokes so much attention. But there is yet little agreement as to whether day-to-day decisions reflect these organizational facts.

Practically every feature in the design of managed care encourages restraint in the use of high-tech and expensive medical interventions. The keystone of the system is the generalist physician, the primary caretaker, whose responsibility it is to serve as gatekeeper between the patient, on the one hand, and the specialist and the technology (the two are intimately linked), on the other. The gatekeeper decides whether the patient's persistent headaches warrant a referral to the neurologist and the CT scan, whether the persistent backaches justify a referral to the orthopedist and the latest imaging machine. To help ensure that generalist physicians do curtail patient access, many managed care organizations structure their contractual relationships with them so as to create financial incentives to keep the gate shut. They adopt a capitation formula, wherein a physician is paid a fixed annual fee for each patient under his care; the fewer times the doctor sees the patient, the more he comes out ahead in time and money. Still more directly, managed care organizations withhold a percentage of the physician's salary, allowing the final sum to depend on overall annual profits and losses.

So physicians who send too many patients to specialists or use too many high-tech procedures may suffer a 20% reduction in income. If they restrict access, they may pocket a 20% increase.[4]

To make still more certain that gatekeepers fulfill their responsibilities, managed care organizations have implemented practice plan formulas that physicians are obliged to follow. HMOs also require participating physicians to obtain formal approval for costly interventions. As one unhappy physician described it, he is forced to call "Debbie in Des Moines" before making a referral or scheduling an expensive test or treatment—and Debbie is primed to say no. To be sure, appeals can be made and often successfully. But physicians are reluctant to take the time and energy to badger their employers, or to become known (on the basis of the company's careful monitoring of their treatment decisions) as outliers who cost the HMO money.[5]

What may be most surprising about these details (surprising, that is, unless one appreciates the staying power of the American Way in health care) is just how well known they are to the public. If ever consumers were alerted to the possible detrimental effects of organizational policies, this is the case! Local newspapers are reporting the sizable salaries and bonuses given to HMO executives. "The total compensation package of the typical health care corporate CEO," reported the *Washington Post*, "was close to $2.9 million last year."[6] They are also turning denials of access into scandal stories, with the HMO presented as a greedy ogre that must be caged. The accounts, written from the perspective of a desperately ill patient seeking an expensive intervention or a longer hospital stay, invariably evoke sympathy for the patient and breed hostility to the distant managed care corporation. Thus, *New York Times* columnist Bob Herbert, in an article entitled "Mugged in the Hospital," asked: "What is a woman supposed to do when, two days after major surgery, her health maintenance organization tells her she must leave the hospital and her physician insists that she stay put?"[7] The *New York Post* ran five consecutive stories under the headline, "HMOs: What You Don't Know Could Kill You." *Glamour* magazine related the story of "Death by HMO." And *Consumer Reports* not only repeated these particular developments but added to them. The photos and captions accompany-

ing its cover story on "How Good Is Your Health Plan?" told of one patient with esophageal cancer who had to wait three months to get an X ray; another patient died from a brain aneurysm apparently because her HMO doctor thought it was a virus and gave her cough syrup.[8]

The stories are so easy to compose that they have become a staple of such popular television programs as *ER*. The heroic doctor alters the medical chart so as not to have to send the asthmatic child across town, as the managed care organization wanted done. In effect, an entire country of patients is being taught to question whether physicians are writing orders to help the patient or to further their company's and their own financial interests.

Not only patients but physicians are exquisitely sensitive to the potential conflicts of interest posed by managed care. Whether this sensitivity will translate into a continuing commitment to putting patients' interests first is unclear, but the tension between professional medical ethics and managed care has been highlighted in almost every major medical journal. The American Medical Association's Council on Ethical and Judicial Affairs in 1990 and then again in 1995 focused attention on the potentially deleterious effects of HMOs' use of bonuses and of withholding of salaries "to make physicians cost conscious . . . [so that] when physicians are deciding whether to order a test, they will recognize that it may have an adverse impact on their income." In the strongest terms, the council inveighs against withholding treatment in order "to preserve the plan's resources. Physicians should not engage in bedside rationing." It also insists that physicians "disclose all available treatment alternatives, regardless of cost, including those potentially beneficial treatments that are not offered under the terms of the plan."[9] Although these injunctions are not enforceable by the AMA, their impact on physicians' behavior may not be trivial.

State legislatures are also becoming very active in the regulation of managed care, generally taking the side of the voter-patient in the design of Patient Protection Acts. In 1995, such acts were introduced into 17 state legislatures. The tempo of activity increased in 1996; in the first six months, according to the patient advocacy group, Families USA, 33 states enacted HMO legislation. "State governments in all regions of the country," noted its report, "often with bipartisan cooperation, are responding to growing

HMO-related complaints by consumers about the care they are not receiving."[10] At least six states, along with Medicare and Medicaid, have prohibited so-called gag rules, wherein managed care organizations do not allow their physicians to inform patients about all possible treatments.[11] So, too, 14 states have barred HMOs from refusing to cover visits to emergency rooms which turned out, upon examination, not to be emergencies, for example, where the patient mistook severe heartburn for a heart attack.[12] Wisconsin is one of a number of states that have enacted regulations that compel HMOs to set time lines for replying to patients' grievances and to accelerate their review of decisions to deny treatment. And some legislatures have begun to consider restricting the percentages of a physician's salary that can be withheld and made dependent upon year-end financial results. Not surprisingly, HMOs are eagerly seeking federal protection from state legislation they consider hostile, claiming that the bills could cost consumers tens of billions of dollars a year.[13]

All the while, a small army of researchers is busily analyzing the impact of managed care on medical decision making. The findings on performance are preliminary—HMO growth is too recent to provide long-term data on morbidity and mortality. But they do suggest that managed care is making strides in fulfilling its mission of reducing the incentives to treatment that characterized fee-for-service medicine. Frequently, although not uniformly, HMOs are also reducing costs for employers; company expenditures for health insurance are growing at a substantially slower pace, according to U. S. Labor Department reports. From July 1, 1995, to June 30, 1996, their costs rose only 0.1%, the smallest increase on record.[14]

In the first instance, the gatekeepers in managed care are relying less heavily upon specialists than their colleagues in fee-for-service.[15] Patients in HMOs experiencing joint pain or chest pain when compared to patients in fee-for-service were "much less likely to be referred to a specialist."[16] HMOs also appear to be using fewer resources when measured by the number of CT scans, Doppler ultrasonograms, cardiac angiography, or coronary artery bypass grafts. The best estimate is of "22 percent fewer procedures, tests, or treatments that were expensive and/or had less costly alternative interventions."[17] So, too, HMOs have reduced, at least somewhat, hospital admissions and length of hospital stays.[18] There is even evidence that HMO patients are experiencing shorter stays in the ICU (which are not under direct HMO control) and are less likely to go on respirators. "The differences," reported one team of investigators, "were quantitatively large, consistent, and often statistically significant. Managed care patients stayed in the ICU, on the average, about 35 percent less time than traditionally insured patients. . . . There was no difference in mortality or ICU readmission rate between the two groups to suggest a benefit from the additional ICU stay of the insured patients." On the other side of the coin, indications are that HMO physicians deliver more preventive care than fee-for-service colleagues. They more frequently screen for hypertension, carry out breast, pelvic, and rectal exams, and promote such health related activities as smoking cessation programs.[19]

What do these specific findings mean in terms of health outcomes? Are HMO patients getting second-rate care? To date, apparently not. In most instances and with the notable exception of mental health, the outcomes for patients are roughly equivalent between HMOs and fee-for-service when congestive heart failure, colon cancer, diabetes, or hypertension are examined.[20] The most notable difference between the two groups is in patient satisfaction. Most respondents to surveys are "reasonably satisfied" with their insurance, whether they are in managed care or fee-for-service. In one poll, for example, 85% of fee-for-service and 78% of managed care groups rated their plans excellent or good. But managed care enrollees are considerably more likely to find fault with one or another aspect of their care; for example, 23% complain about access to specialty care, as against 8% in fee-for-service; similar differences mark their answers to questions about choice of physicians or waiting time for appointments.[21] So, too, HMO patients rate the interpersonal aspects of the relationship with their physicians lower than those in fee-for-service; the physicians spend less time with them and seem less concerned about them.[22] However, when the questions focus on cost, the HMO respondents seem more pleased and report savings on out-of-pocket expenses.[23]

For the moment, it is a draw overall. To be sure, this conclusion may reflect too little research, too short a time span, or too crude a method of measurement. Perhaps American medicine was so bloated with interventions that a 22% cutback did not have a negative impact. We may also know too little about when to carry out highly invasive interventions, like angiography, or how to measure quality of care with precision. Or the results may be testimony to the fact that outsiders are monitoring HMOs so carefully that they are preventing a decline in quality of care. Perhaps the HMOs themselves are behaving responsibly because they are new; as they try to build up a membership base, they remain anxious about competition, do not want to lose employer confidence, are wary about adverse publicity, and are fearful of large malpractice losses. Perhaps they are so new that there has not yet been time for corporate raiders or even Mafia-type organizations to take them over. Possibly, too, physicians are taking ethics to heart and elevating patient well-being over personal income. Patients, for their part, may be successfully badgering HMOs into giving them the treatment choices that they want, not taking no for an answer and getting access to quasi-experimental therapies (like bone marrow transplant for advanced breast cancer) and very expensive ones (like organ transplantation). At the same time, HMOs may be benefiting from the fact that their enrollees tend to be younger and healthier than patients in fee-for-service; this epidemiological fact may be obscuring the long-term negative impact of managed care. There is some evidence for each of these propositions, but in all events, the dire predictions of critics are not being realized, or, more cautiously put, have not yet been realized. What the system will look like ten years hence when HMOs have lost their novelty and are no longer the object of such intense scrutiny is truly anybody's guess.[24]

Finally, in this state of suspense, what are the implications of managed care for national health insurance? If middle-class Americans are giving up some of their dedication to have all the medicine they want, at least at the margins and under some duress, is there a prospect that the United States will abandon its outlier position and realize health insurance for all by the year 2020? For the moment, there is little reason for optimism. The bills that work their way through Congress almost uniformly maintain the hegemony of private insurance companies over health care. They restrict insurance companies' more egregious discriminatory practices, in the process making it easier for employees to carry insurance with them from job to job and to provide them with protection against discrimination on the basis of pre-existing medical conditions. Congressional enactment of a pilot program of tax-free medical savings accounts also reflects a desire to serve the interests of the middle classes, but no one else's. Thus there appears to be no immediate prospect of massive government intervention on behalf of the millions who earn too little to purchase their own health insurance. Indeed, the enthusiasm with which the "end to welfare as we know it" has recently been greeted suggests just how unlikely such a prospect is.

The only qualification to this conclusion comes from the recent experiments with using managed care organizations to treat Medicaid and, in some cases, Medicare patients. Were costs of health care to drop dramatically, a national health insurance program might become feasible. But even here, there are cautions. If special managed care programs are initiated that serve only the poor, they are very likely to provide substandard treatment. There is already some evidence for this proposition in the existing plans. Moreover, we know from the past that programs that served only the poor inevitably became poor programs.[25]

In the end, the agenda that will occupy the United States for at least the next decade is whether managed care itself can meet enough of the middle-class demand for access to technology and at the same time contain costs. Only after that issue is resolved is it likely that attention will turn to the underprivileged. One can imagine a scenario in which HMOs deliver just that modicum of medicine to the middle classes which is effective and efficient, thereby reining in costs. At that moment, the predicament that brought about the demise of the Clinton plan, the need to simultaneously expand coverage and restrict costs, to increase access and to ration, would disappear. Once the medical needs of the middle classes were met in a way that satisfied both them and the Congressional Budget Office, the federal government might be able to meet the needs of others. But that scenario is a distant one and each of the steps along the way remains highly problematic.

Notes

INTRODUCTION

1. For a very perceptive discussion of the theme of American exceptionalism, and an objection to it, see Theda Skocpol, *Protecting Soldiers and Mothers* (Cambridge, Mass.: Harvard University Press, 1992), 15–23.
2. Quoted by Paul Starobin, "Flunking Economics," *National Journal*, March 12, 1994, 586.
3. Robert D. Putnam, *Making Democracy Work* (Princeton, N.J.: Princeton University Press, 1993), 8.

CHAPTER ONE

1. Jerome L. Schwartz, "Early History of Prepaid Medical Care Plans," *Bulletin of the History of Medicine*, 39 (1965), 450–53.
2. For an insightful history of Blue Cross which focuses on New York but takes the story well beyond that, see the essays in the *Journal of Health Politics, Policy and Law*, 16 (1991). This special issue of the *Journal* was under the guest editorship of Daniel M. Fox, David Rosner, and Rosemary A. Stevens, and was entitled, "Between Public and Private: A Half Century of Blue Cross and Blue Shield in New York" (hereafter "Between Public and Private"). An early version of this chapter also appears there. For the numbers and growth of Blue Cross, see the essay therein by Lawrence D. Brown, "Capture and Culture: Organizational Identity in New York Blue Cross," 658–59.
3. Robert Padgug, "Looking Backward: Empire Blue Cross and Blue Shield as an Object of Historical Analysis," in "Between Public and Private," 799.
4. Louis Reed, *Blue Cross and Medical Service Plans* (Washington, D.C.: Federal Security Agency, October 1947), 28, 69.
5. Herman Miles Somers and Anne Ramsay Somers, *Doctors, Patients, and Health Insurance* (Washington, D.C.: Brookings Institution, 1961), 369.
6. Frank Van Dyk, "Experience Reveals the Worth of Group Hospitalization" (delivered at the New England Hospital Association Conference, Boston,

February 16, 1934), 13. The Van Dyk materials are part of the Empire Blue Cross and Blue Shield Archives, New York City (hereafter, Blue Cross Archives). In keeping with its not-for-profit status, Blue Cross was unwilling to adopt the alternative model of commercial insurance companies, such as Metropolitan Life, who organized a network of salesmen that worked to enroll subscribers on a commission basis.

7. New York State Group Plan Directors, minutes of meeting of January 29, 1938, in Davis Papers, New York Academy of Medicine, New York.

8. Annual Report for the Director of Hospital Service Plan Commission, American Hospital Association, 1943, in United Medical Service History File, "Public Education," 15–18, Blue Cross Archives.

9. Ibid., 15.

10. *Oil, Chemical and Atomic Union News*, August 5, 1957.

11. E. A. Van Steenwyk (executive vice president of AHS of Philadelphia), "Why Blue Cross Must Advertise," 1958, p. 34, Davis Papers.

12. "Every 40 Seconds," January 24, 1944, WNYC, in the Pink Papers, Blue Cross Archives.

13. *Brooklyn Times-Union*, April 22, 1935.

14. Rosanne Amberson, "Hospital Care at Three Cents a Day," *The Forecast*, June 1935, 247–48.

15. Although Blue Cross did not itself make the point, some observers noted that if not for the plan, the public hospital system would have been overburdened. The plan was, therefore, performing an important civic function, rescuing the municipality from added costs and an extraordinary burden. See the editorial in the *New York Times*, March 3, 1939, "Hospitals and Doctors." Note, too, the speech of Newbold Morris, as reported in the *New York Times*, March 18, 1939, to the effect that the voluntary hospitals had 6500 empty beds while the public hospital system was operating at 95% of capacity.

16. Josephine Pearson, "The Luxury of Illness," *New York Woman*, January 1, 1937, 9–10. Van Dyk released a similar letter to the press: "I had just as good care as I had formerly, when I was paying full price." (*White Plains Reporter*, July 9, 1937.)

17. See, for example, *New York Times*, April 4, 1933: "State Physicians Score Wilbur Plan," and advocate a "limited form of hospitalization insurance."

18. Clipping of a New York newspaper, unidentified, of May 1935, in Blue Cross Archive. See also *New York Times* and *New York Tribune* of February 19, 1938.

19. Quoted in the *Bridgeport Herald*, August 8, 1938.

20. *New York Times*, July 22, 1937, November 2, 1940; *New York Tribune*, November 2, 1940.

21. Paul Starr, *The Social Transformation of American Medicine* (New York: Basic Books, 1982), 280.

22. Blue Cross, Associated Hospital Services, *Annual Report for 1942*, Blue Cross Archives.

23. Blue Cross, Associated Hospital Services, *Annual Report for 1942*, 13,17, Blue Cross Archives.

24. Blue Cross, Associated Hospital Services, *Annual Report for 1942*, 2–6.

25. Blue Cross, Associated Hospital Services, *Annual Report for 1943*, "A Timely Message."

26. Leo Wirz, Jr., to Louis Pink, February 16, 1949; Louis Pink to Leo Wirz, Jr., February 18, 1949, Pink Papers, New York Academy of Medicine.

27. Louis Pink, radio broadcast of February 3, 1946, 3; transcript in the Pink Papers, Blue Cross Archives.

28. *Blue Cross Bulletin*, 11 (1948), 1.

29. E. Dwight Barnett, "The Impact of Blue Cross Public Relations on the Political Scene," *Hospital Council Bulletin*, May 1948, 13–17, in the Davis Papers. It was again reprinted in *Hospital Management* in June 1948. Barnett was director of the Harper Hospital in Detroit, Michigan, and the text of the article was originally delivered as a talk before the Joint Conference of Blue Cross Hospital Plans and Hospital Representatives of the Tri-State Hospital Assembly, May 5, 1948.

30. Abraham Oseroff, "Blue Cross–Blue Shield and Free Enterprise," File A-4, Davis Papers, New York Academy of Medicine.

31. Rufus Rorem, quoted in *Hospitals*, February 1944, clipping in the Davis Papers, New York Academy of Medicine; Roy Larson, "Management's Interest in Employees' Health," speech to a Blue Cross Conference, New York, October 30, 1945, Blue Cross Archives.

32. See Pink's remarks, for example, in the Blue Cross, Associated Hospital Services, *Annual Report of December 31, 1949* (January 31, 1950), on the need for government to "care for those who cannot pay."

33. See the Blue Cross, Associated Hospital Service, *Annual Reports of 1947, 1948, and 1949*. The opening two pages of each report address the inflation issues. The quotation on commercial insurance is from the report of 1951, 3.

34. Brief for Associated Hospital Services of New York: Application for Rate Increase, Davis Papers, File A-1, New York Academy of Medicine.

35. J. Walter Thompson, minutes of meeting, November 3, 1961, J. Walter Thompson Inc., New York City.

36. J. Walter Thompson, minutes of meeting, October 23, 1961, J. Walter Thompson Inc., New York City.

37. As Charles Garside, chairman and president of the board of directors, summed it up in the Blue Cross, Associated Hospital Services, *Annual Report for 1958*, 3. "The demands of labor, the growing use of hospital facilities, and the almost fantastically rapid advances in medical science will cause hospital costs to increase, notwithstanding economies achieved through improved hospital administration."

38. Social Research Inc., "Consumer Attitudes toward Blue Cross and Blue Shield," 4–6, Colman Papers, Box A5, Blue Cross Archives.

39. Ibid., 6.

CHAPTER TWO

1. Howard Markel, "The Genesis of the Iron Lung," *Archives of Pediatrics & Adolescent Medicine*, 148 (1994), 1174–76.

2. Philip Drinker and Louis A. Shaw, "An Apparatus for the Prolonged Administration of Artificial Respiration," *Journal of Clinical Investigation*, 7 (1929), 229–47. For a general history of the American encounter with polio, see John R. Paul, *A History of Poliomyelitis* (New Haven, Conn.: Yale University Press, 1971). For a defense of the machine against Lewis Thomas's denigration of it as a "halfway technology," see James H. Maxwell, "The Iron Lung: Halfway Technology or Necessary Step?" *Milbank Quarterly*, 64 (1986), 3–29.

3. Quoted in Markel, "The Genesis of the Iron Lung," 1176.

4. Philip Drinker and Louis Agassiz Shaw, "The Prolonged Administration of Artificial Respiration," *Journal of the Franklin Institute*, 213 (1932), 336.

5. *New York Medical Week*, 9 (1929), August 17, 1929 (11); 10 (1931), August 29, 1931, (11); September 19, 1931 (9). City of New York, Department of Health, *Weekly Bulletin*, 18 (1929), 220.

6. James L. Wilson, "Respiratory Failure in Poliomyelitis," *American Journal of Diseases of Children*, 43 (1932), 1433–53; Irving J. Sands, "Practical Considerations in the Diagnosis and Treatment of Poliomyelitis," *New York State Journal of Medicine*, 34 (1934), 587–90.

7. John Fitch Landon, "An Analysis of 88 Cases of Poliomyelitis Treated in the Drinker Respirator," *Journal of Pediatrics*, 5 (1934), 3–5.

8. Murray B. Gordon, "Poliomyelitis," *New York State Journal of Medicine*, 32 (1932), 1366.

9. Bernard Charles Hecht, "Survey of Anterior Poliomyelitis," *Medical Journal and Record*, 135 (1932), 24.

10. Conrad Wesselhoeft, "Respiratory Failure in Acute Poliomyelitis," *NEJM*, 228 (1943), 561.

11. British Medical Research Council, "Breathing Machines and Their Use in Treatment," London, 1939 (New York Academy of Medicine collection), 27.

12. The story is told most fully by Leonard Hawkins with Milton Lomask, *The Man in the Iron Lung* (New York: Doubleday & Company, 1956).

13. Anne Walters and Jim Marugg, *Beyond Endurance* (New York: Harper & Row, 1954); Hawkins, *The Man in the Iron Lung*; Gene Roehling, "I Live in an Iron Lung," *Saturday Evening Post*, March 24, 1951, 26.

14. David L. Sills, *The Volunteers: Means and Ends in a National Organization* (Glencoe, Ill.: Free Press, 1957), 135–37.

15. Leo Mayer to Basil O'Connor, June 30, 1939, in the files of the NFIP, located in the March of Dimes Archives, Mt. Vernon, New York.

16. James L. Wilson to Dr. Don W. Gudakunst, May 1, 1941. On the "coffin-like" point, see his letter to O'Connor, June 20, 1941, March of Dimes Archives.

17. Morris Fishbein to Basil O'Connor, July 21, 1941, March of Dimes Archives.

18. Wilson's memorandum: "Michigan Respirator Survey for Poliomyelitis," April 9, 1942, 1, in the March of Dimes Archives.

19. Wilson had a third agenda, which we will not be treating here: The NFIP should help to develop a respirator jacket that would enclose only the chest, thereby rendering home care and even hospital care more practical and less frightening.

20. British Medical Research Council, "Breathing Machines," 6.

21. Philip Drinker, Thomas J. Shaugnessy, and Douglas P. Murray, "The Drinker Respirator," *JAMA*, 95 (1930), 1252.

22. James L. Wilson to Dr. Don W. Gudakunst, August 24, 1940, 1, in "The Suggested Program for the National Foundation For Infantile Paralysis in Handling the Respiratory Problem in Poliomyelitis." March of Dimes Archives.

23. Lee Schmid to Dr. Kenneth Landauer, February 7, 1949, 1, March of Dimes Archives. For a typical public statement, see Joseph G. Molner, "Complete Care of Infantile Paralysis Patients Demands Organization of the Community," *Hospitals*, 20 (1946), 40–41.

24. George P. Voss to state representatives, August 12, 1949, March of Dimes Archives.

25. Naomi Rogers, *Dirt and Disease: Polio before FDR* (New Brunswick, N.J.: Rutgers University Press, 1992), 174.

26. Tony Gould, *A Summer Plague: Polio and Its Survivors* (New Haven, Conn.: Yale University Press, 1995), 81. The year before, however, the rates were much closer — 1.7 for whites, and 2.1 for blacks.

27. NFIP, "Doctor . . . What Can I Do? Facts about Infantile Paralysis," 2nd ed. (New York: NFIP, 1942), 10, March of Dimes Archives. Naomi Rogers makes clear that this middle-class predominance was not always true for the disease. In the Progressive era, polio was more prevalent in ghetto slums than middle class neighborhoods (*Dirt and Disease*, 1, 47–49).

28. The pamphlet was published in 1942 and is in the collection of the New York Academy of Medicine.

29. "A New Weapon Against Polio," NFIP Release, 1, March of Dimes Archives.

30. Memorandum of October 25, 1950, no name, March of Dimes Archives. The NFIP was occasionally called upon to supply iron lungs for other than polio patients, and here, too, it responded with one eye on need and the other on image. In setting up a storage facility with a New York City ambulance company, the NFIP noted the advantage of having a number of machines so near an air-

port with national connections. Moreover, New York City generated a large number of emergency calls: "A couple were not for polio patients, but the persons requesting the aid, especially the police forces, were those with whom we should cooperate." And NFIP officials noted, "This cooperation paid off, as recent as this year's March of Dimes [campaign appeal] during which time we had occasion to seek police permission for parking the Mobile Field Service Unit. This, of course, brings up a question as to whether or not we may use our equipment for other than polio emergencies. Reciprocity, however, dictates our action in this regard." (Lee Schmid to Dr. Kenneth Landauer, February 7, 1949, March of Dimes Archives.)

31. Memorandum of July 19, 1958, NFIP files, no name or recipient noted, March of Dimes Archives.

32. Lee Schmid to Dr. H. Van Riper, May 28, 1949, 3.

33. Hawkins, *The Man in the Iron Lung*, 20, 173–75.

34. Anne Walters and Jim Marugg, *Beyond Endurance* (New York: Harper & Row, 1954), 13, 21, 43–45, 62, 173–74.

35. Lawrence Alexander, *The Iron Cradle* (New York: Crowell, 1954), 22, 33, 42, 46, 177–79, 185.

36. See Sheila M. Rothman, *Living in the Shadow of Death* (New York: Basic Books, 1994).

37. Kenneth S. Landauer, "Respirator Centers," March 8, 1951, 1, March of Dimes Archives.

38. Press release of the NFIP, February 3, 1952, 3, March of Dimes Archives.

39. "Annual Statistical Report of Respirator Centers—1952" and "Annual Statistical Report of Respiratory Centers—1953," NFIP files, March of Dimes Archives.

40. "Introduction," to a memo, 1953, 3, March of Dimes Archives. In 1954, the NFIP found that of the 1500 polio patients using respirators, the great majority were still scattered in over 300 hospitals around the country. (Eighty percent of these hospitals had three or fewer such patients.)

41. Herbert J. Seddon, "Economic Aspects of the Management of Poliomyelitis," International Poliomyelitis Conference, *Papers and Discussions* (Philadelphia: Lippincott, 1948), 35.

42. Chester S. Keefer, "Social Aspects of Poliomyelitis: United States," Third International Poliomyelitis Conference, *Papers and Discussions* (Philadelphia: Lippincott, 1955), 16.

43. Nathaniel W. Faxon, "General Hospitals Have the Responsibility," *Hospitals*, 20 (1946), 44, 47.

44. Hart E. Van Riper, Letter to the Editor, *Journal of the American Medical Association*, 141 (1949), 1260; "Polio Fee Schedule Adopted," *Journal of the Tennessee State Medical Association*, 42 (1949), 13–14.

CHAPTER THREE

1. For one notable exception to the benign interpretations of the Medicare strategy, see Lawrence Jacobs, in *The Health of Nations* (Ithaca, New York: Cornell University Press, 1993), 161. Jacobs comes closest to the position I present here when he writes: "In pursuit of what was supposed to be the means (Medicare), reformers effectively sacrificed their long-term objectives by deliberately, even eagerly, designing Medicare to prevent the program's future development."

2. James Morone, *The Democratic Wish* (New York: Basic Books, 1990).

3. Paul Starr, *The Social Transformation of American Medicine* (New York: Basic Books, 1982), Book Two.

4. See, for example, John Ikenberry and Theda Skocpol, "The Political Formation of the American Welfare State in Historical and Comparative Perspective," *Comparative Social Research*, 6 (1983), 87–148.

5. Jacobs, *Health of Nations*, 139.

6. U.S. Congress, House of Representatives, Hearings before the Committee on Ways and Means, "Medical Care for the Aged," 1963, Part I, 27.

7. Hearings, Part I, 28.

8. Hearings, Part I, 54.

9. Hearings, Part I, 27.

10. Hearings, Part III, 621.

11. Hearings, Part I, 37.

12. Hearings, Part II, 297.

13. Hearings, Part II, 645–46.

14. Hearings, Part II, 295.

15. Hearings, Part I, 257.

16. Hearings, Part III, 1269.

17. Hearings, Part II, 257.

18. Hearings, Part I, 29.

19. Hearings, Part II, 305.

20. Hearings, Part III, 623.

21. Hearings, Part I, 28.

22. Hearings, Part I, 36.

23. As quoted in Jacobs, *Health of Nations*, 105.

24. Hearings, Part III, 1652.

25. Hearings, Part III, 1653.

26. Hearings, Part III, 1654.

27. Hearings, Part II, 1652–54.

28. Hearings, Part III, 1569–70.

29. Hearings, Part III, 1416.

30. Hearings, Part I, 31.

31. Hearings, Part I, 37, 119.

32. Hearings, Part II, 257.

33. Hearings, Part III, 1292

34. Hearings, Part III, 1440.

35. Hearings, Part II, 284.

36. Hearings, Part III, 1292

37. Hearings, Part I, 551.

38. Hearings, Part II, 333.

39. Hearings, Part I, 31.

40. Hearings, Part I, 31.

41. Hearings, Part III, 1293, 1587.

42. Hearings, Part I, 159.

43. Jacobs, *Health of Nations*, 162.

44. Jacobs, *Health of Nations*, 213. The point was first made by Theodore Marmor in *The Politics of Medicare* (Chicago: Aldine, 1970).

CHAPTER FOUR

1. William J. Kolff, "Birth, Adolescence, and Maturity of the Artificial Kidney," transcript of a lecture in "Proceedings of the Conference to Consider the Treatment of Patients with Chronic Kidney Disease with Uremia," 31–33 (on file at the National Kidney Disease Foundation); Richard A. Rettig, "End-Stage Renal Disease and the 'Cost' of Medical Technology" (Rand Paper Series, October 1977) 2–4.

2. Rettig, "End-Stage Renal Disease," 5–7. Rettig, who has written extensively and wisely on ESRD policy, based his account on an interview with Scribner.

3. Drummond Rennie, R. A. Rettig, and A. J. Wing, "Limited Resources and the Treatment of End-Stage Renal Failure in Britain and the United States," *Quarterly Journal of Medicine*, 56 (1985), 322–26; Richard A. Rettig, "The Federal Government and Social Planning for End-Stage Renal Disease," *Seminars in Nephrology*, 2 (1982), 116.

4. *Newsweek*, June 11, 1962, 92.

5. Belding Scribner, "Current Patterns of Operation of a Community Dialysis Center," reported in "Proceedings of the Conference to Consider the Treatment of Patients with Chronic Kidney Disease with Uremia," 43.

6. Rettig, "The Federal Government and Social Planning for End-Stage Renal Disease," 117.

7. David S. David, "The Agony and Ecstasy of the Nephrologist," Letters to the Editor, JAMA, 222 (1972), 584–85; Harry S. Abram, "The Psychiatrist, the Treatment of Chronic Renal Failure, and the Prolongation of Life: II," *American Journal of Psychiatry*, 126 (1969), 46–47; R. A. Gutman, W. W. Stead and R. R.

Robinson, "Physical Activity and Employment Status of Patients on Maintenance Dialysis," *NEJM*, 304 (1981), 309–13; Jonathan Cummings, "Hemodialysis — Feelings, Facts, Fantasies," *American Journal of Nursing*, 70 (1970), 70–76.

8. *NAPH News*, Special Anniversary Issue, 4 (1973), 22.

9. Abram, "The Psychiatrist, the Treatment of Chronic Renal Failure, and the Prolongation of Life: II," 162–63.

10. Richard A. Rettig and Norman G. Levinsky, *Kidney Failure and the Federal Government* (Washington, D.C.: National Academy Press, Institute of Medicine, 1991), 65.

11. American Medical Association and National Kidney Foundation, "Proceedings, Conference to Consider the Treatment of Patients with Chronic Kidney Disease with Uremia," New York City, June 20–22, 1963, 67. See also, Richard A. Rettig, "Origins of the Medicare Kidney Disease Entitlement," K. E. Hanna, ed., *Biomedical Politics* (Washington, D.C.: National Academy Press, Institute of Medicine, 1991), 176–208.

12. Rettig, "The Federal Government and Social Planning," 111, 119.

13. As quoted by Carl Gottschalk in his testimony before the U. S. Senate, United States Senate, *Hearings before the Subcommittee on Health of the Committee on Labor and Public Welfare*, 91st Congress, 2nd session, on H.R. 3355, February 17–18, 1970, 159.

14. *NAPH News*, 1 (1969), 1–2; "The Kidney Care Issue," *Hospital Practice*, April 1973, 49.

15. *NAPH News*, 11 (1972), 6.

16. Institute of Medicine, *Kidney Failure*, 65. Later, as we shall see, the age of dialysis patients, as well as their social class, will change.

17. *NAPH News*, 3 (1972), 1.

18. See the reports by these groups in *NAPH News*, 3 (1970), 5–6.

19. *NAPH News*, 2 (1971), 8.

20. See United States Senate, *Hearings before the Subcommittee on Health of the Committee on Labor and Public Welfare*, 91st Congress, 2nd session, on H.R. 3355, February 17–18, 1970 (hereafter, 1970 Senate Hearings). See also House of Representatives Ways and Means Committee, *Hearings on National Health Proposals*, Part 7, November 4, 1971, 1524–2229 (hereafter, House Hearings, 1971). For 1972, see United States Senate, *Hearings before the Subcommittee on the Handicapped of the Committee on Labor and Public Welfare*, 92nd Congress, 2nd session, on H.R. 8395, May 15, 18, 23, 1972 (hereafter, Senate Hearings, 1972). On Public Law 62-903, see the *Congressional Record*, 92nd Congress, 2nd Session, vol. 118, 33003–33009 (hereafter, *Congressional Record*, 1972).

21. David Sanders and Jessie Dukeminier, Jr., "Medical Advance and Legal Lag," *UCLA Law Review*, 15 (1968), 357–413.

22. David, "The Agony and Ecstasy," 584–85.

23. Senate Hearings, 1972, 334–35.

24. Senate Hearings, 1970, 192.

25. *Congressional Record*, 1972, 33004–7.

26. Institute of Medicine, *Kidney Failure*, 65.

27. *Congressional Record*, 1972, 33004.

28. Senate Hearings, 1970, 118, 156; House Hearings, 1971, 1525.

29. Senate Hearings, 1970, 192–93.

30. Senate Hearings, 1970, 117, 121.

31. House Hearings, 1971, 1540–43.

32. House Hearing, 1971, 1545–56.

33. *New York Times*, September 3, 1972.

34. *New York Times*, October 18, 1972: Roslyn Barreaux, "Family Fund Gives Kidney Patients Machines and Help."

35. *Newsweek*, July 26, 1971, 51.

36. Undated announcement (1969), announcing the formation of NAPH; *NAPH News*, 1 (1969), 3.

37. Senate Hearings, 1972, 413.

38. House Hearings, 1971, 2228.

39. *Congressional Record*, 1972, 33008.

40. Institute of Medicine, *Kidney Failure*, 32, 65.

41. Published by the Brookings Institution, Washington, D.C., 1984. Quotations from 33, 113, 135.

42. Richard J. Margolis, "Cost per Life: $22,000," *New York Times*, March 8, 1991, A29

CHAPTER FIVE

1. Henrik H. Bendixen and John M. Kinney, "History of Intensive Care," chapter 1 in American College of Surgeons, *Manual of Surgical Intensive Care* (Philadelphia: American College of Surgeons, 1977), 3–14. J. D. Young and M. K. Sykes, "Artificial Ventilation: History, Equipment and Techniques," *Thorax*, 45 (1990), 753–58; L. H. Hawkins, "The Experimental Development of Modern Resuscitation," *Resuscitation* 1 (1972), 9–24; Thomas L. Petty, "The Modern Evolution of Mechanical Ventilation," *Clinics in Chest Medicine*, 9 (1988), 1–10; Mark Hilberman, "The Evolution of Intensive Care Units," *Critical Care Medicine*, 3 (1975), 159–65.

2. Gordon L. Snider, "Historical Perspective on Mechanical Ventilation: From Simple Life Support to Ethical Dilemma," *American Review of Respiratory Diseases*, 140 (1982), S4–5.

3. For an overview of the Quinlan story and citations to the vast literature, see David J. Rothman, *Strangers at the Bedside* (New York: Basic Books, 1991), chapter 8.

4. An earlier version of this analysis of bioethics and rationing appeared in the *New York Review of Books*, "Rationing Life," David J. Rothman, February 1992. Daniel Callahan, *Setting Limits: Medical Goals in an Aging Society* (New York: Simon & Schuster, 1987).

5. Daniel Callahan, *What Kind of Life: The Limits of Medical Progress* (New York: Simon & Schuster, 1990), 19, 26–27, 35, 40, 66.

6. Ibid., 110, 121, 127–29, 139.

7. Ibid., 200–207.

8. John F. Kilner, *Who Lives? Who Dies?* (New Haven, Conn.: Yale University Press, 1990), 3.

9. Paul T. Menzel, *Strong Medicine: The Ethical Rationing of Health Care* (New York: Oxford University Press, 1990), viii.

10. Kilner, *Who Lives? Who Dies?* chapter 19.

11. Menzel, *Strong Medicine*, 14.

12. Menzel, *Strong Medicine*, 195–200.

13. I do not want to leave the impression that bioethicists speak with one voice on rationing. For example, Samuel Gorovitz, in *Drawing the Line* (New York: Oxford University Press, 1991), 80, notes that addressing questions about how to ration can become a "destructive" exercise, "for to answer them at all, even on the most tentative basis, is to devalue entire categories of people. . . . Until we are unable to avoid them, it may be best to keep on trying."

14. Troyen A. Brennan, *Just Doctoring: Medical Ethics in the Liberal State* (Los Angeles: University of California Press, 1991), 177–97.

15. J. E. Zimmerman, D. P. Wagner, W. A. Knaus et al., "The Use of Risk Predictions to Identify Candidates for Intermediate Care Units. Implications for Intensive Care Utilization and Costs," *Chest*, 108 (1995), 490–99.

16. Philip Roth, *Patrimony: A True Story* (New York: Simon & Schuster, 1991), 232.

17. Andrew Malcolm, *Someday* (New York: Alfred Knopf, 1991), 289.

18. Derek Humphry, *Final Exit: The Practicalities of Self-Deliverance and Assisted Suicide for the Dying* (New York: Carol Publishing, 1991).

19. Daniel M. Fox and Howard M. Leichter, "Rationing Care in Oregon: The New Accountability," and Lawrence D. Brown, "The National Politics of Oregon's Rationing Plan," *Health Affairs*, 10 (1991), 7–51; Charles J. Dougherty, "Setting Health Care Priorities: Oregon's Next Steps," *Hastings Center Report*, 21 (1991), Conference Report, 1–10.

CHAPTER SIX

1. Lest anyone in the White House miss these findings, the foundations sponsoring the polls sent the results directly to Ira Magaziner, head of the president's

Task Force on Health Care Reform. See, for example, Martila and Kiley Inc. and the Harvard School of Public Health, "Strategic Observations from a Robert Wood Johnson Survey on American Attitudes toward Health Care Reform," April 23, 1993, 26–27, Box 3305, Task Force Papers at the National Archives (hereafter cited as Task Force Papers).

2. Mollyann Brodie and Robert J. Blendon, "The Public's Contribution to Congressional Gridlock on Health Care Reform," *Journal of Health Politics, Policy, and Law*, 20 (1995), 403–5.

3. Jennifer N. Edwards, Robert J. Blendon, and Robert Leitman, "The Worried Middle Class," chapter 4 in Blendon and Tracey Stelzer Hyams, eds., *Reforming the System*, (New York: Faulkner and Gray, 1992).

4. Ibid., 290–92.

5. Haynes Johnson and David S. Broder, *The System* (Boston: Little, Brown, 1996), 60. The credit may have been misplaced, the authors note, but the Democrats were convinced that they had found "a powerful issue to use against President George Bush."

6. Sven Steinmo and Jon Watts, "It's the Institutions Stupid," *Journal of Health Politics, Policy and Law*, 20 (1995), 362.

7. Brodie and Blendon, "The Public's Contribution," 403.

8. Theda Skocpol, *Boomerang* (New York: W. W. Norton, 1996), 178.

9. See the memo of Paul Starr, March 22, 1993, entitled "Karen Davis's 'Alternative Model,'" 5, Box 3305, Task Force Papers.

10. Paul Starr to Ira Magaziner, memorandum of February 7, 1993, Box 3308, Task Force Papers.

11. Walter Zelman to Ira Magaziner, January 16 [1993], Box 3308, Task Force Papers.

12. Walter Zelman to Bob Boorstin, March 10 [1993], Box 3308, Task Force Papers.

13. See the February 21, 1993, memo in the Task Force Files, Box 3305.

14. Paul Starobin, "Flunking Economics?" *National Journal*, 26, (March 12, 1994), 581.

15. Paul Starr, *The Logic of Health Care Reform* (New York: Whittle Books in Association with Penguin Books, 1994), 42.

16. Ibid., 44–45

17. Ibid., 46.

18. Walter Zelman, "The Rationale Behind the Clinton Health Care Reform Plan," *Health Affairs*, 13 (1994), 21–22.

19. The material was compiled by the Center for Intramural Research at the Agency for Health Care Policy and Research of the Department of Health and Human Services. See Box 3309 of the Task Force Papers; quotations are from pages 1, 16, 25.

20. See "Briefing Book: Ethics," Box 2274, Task Force Papers.

21. Group 317, April 7, 1993, "Personal Memorandum: Issues Paper," Box 3308, Task Force Papers.

22. Jack Hadley and Stephen Zuckerman, "Health Reform: The Good, the Bad, and the Bottom Line," *Health Affairs*, 13 (1994), 118–19.

23. Mark Pauly, "The Clinton Plan: What Happened to the Tough Choices?" *Health Affairs*, 13 (1994), 147.

24. Quoted by Nat Hentoff, "Health Rationing," *Washington Post*, February 19, 1994, A27.

25. Henry Aaron, "Sowing the Seeds of Reform in 1994," *Health Affairs*, 13 (1994), 58, 64–65.

26. Victor Fuchs, "The Clinton Plan: A Researcher Examines Reform," *Health Affairs*, 13 (1994), 112–13.

27. Allen D. Verhey, "The Health Security Act," cover story for the *Christian Century*, January 26, 1994.

28. Robert J. Blendon, Mollyann Brodie, and John Benson, "What Happened to Americans' Support for the Clinton Health Plan?" *Health Affairs*, 14 (1995), 9–11.

29. Martila and Kiley Inc. and the Harvard School of Public Health, "Strategic Observations from a Robert Wood Johnson Survey on American Attitudes toward Health Care Reform," April 23, 1993, 26–27, Box 3305, Task Force Papers. See also Daniel Yankelovich, "The Debate That Wasn't: The Public and the Clinton Plan," *Health Affairs*, 14 (1995), 13.

30. The headline from a *Time* magazine story captures the spirit well: "What You're Not Being Told," February 14, 1994, 22.

31. Mark Turnbull, "US States Seek a 'Reality Check' on Health Plan," *Christian Science Monitor*, September 21, 1993, 1.

32. John W. Kennedy, "Rx for America," *Christianity Today*, April 25, 1994, 38ff.

33. Federal Document Clearing House, Congressional Testimony, May 3, 1994; Bureau of National Affairs, "Clinton Plan Would Cut in Half Uncompensated Care Costs for U.S. Firms," *Washington Insider*, April 20, 1994.

34. Quoted by Alfred G. Haggerty, "California Anti-Single-Payer Drive Revs Up," *National Underwriter, Life and Health/Financial Services Edition*, June 6, 1994.

35. *USA Today*, October 6, 1993, 13A.

36. Quotations by David Cannella, "Health-Care Ethics: Who Plays God?" *Arizona Republic*, September 26, 1993, A1.

37. Testimony of Paul Malek before the Social Security Subcommittee of the House Ways and Means Committee, Federal Information Systems, Federal News Service, February 23, 1994.

38. Nat Hentoff, "Health Rationing," *Washington Post*, February 19, 1994, A27.

39. "Senior Group Raises Health Care Alarm," *Rocky Mountain News*, April 11, 1994.

40. "Health Care Reform Raises Questions of Individual Rights," *Christian Science Monitor*, March 29, 1994.

41. Elizabeth McCaughey, "No Exit," *New Republic*, February 7, 1994, 22–25.

42. "Media in the Middle: Fairness and Accuracy in the 1994 Health Care Reform Debate," a report by the Annenberg Public Policy Center of the University of Pennsylvania, February 1995, 17–19.

43. Lise Deitsch Taylor, "Managing Liability in Managed Care," *New Jersey Law Journal*, November 8, 1993, 3.

44. George M. Kraw, "Medical Rationing," *Legal Times*, December 27, 1993, 30; Nat Hentoff, "Health Rationing," *Washington Post*, February 19, 1994, A27.

45. C. Everett Koop, "Letter," *Medical Economics*, 12 (1994), January Special Issue on "The State of Health Care in America," 4.

EPILOGUE

1. *Wall Street Journal*, August 2, 1996, 28; Dana Gelb Safran, Alvin R. Tarlov, and William H. Rogers, "Primary Care Performance in Fee-for-Service and Prepaid Health Care Systems," *JAMA*, 271 (1994), 1579.

2. Robert H. Miller and Harold S. Luft, "Managed Care Plan Performance Since 1980," *JAMA*, 271 (1994), 1512.

3. Lawrence Jacobs, "Politics of American Supply State: Health Reform and Technology," *Health Affairs*, 14 (1995), 155.

4. According to Marsha Gold et al., between 50% and 75% of HMOs use financial incentives to reduce interventions. Some three-quarters of the HMOs also used practice guidelines. ("A National Survey of the Arrangements Managed-Care Plans Make with Physicians," *NEJM*, 333 (1995), 1680.)

5. For one study showing that physicians are proving to be responsive to these measures, see Eve A. Kerr et al., "Managed Care and Capitation in California," *Annals of Internal Medicine*, 123 (1995), 500–504.

6. Stuart Auerbach, "Managed Care Backlash," *Washington Post*, June 25, 1996, Z12.

7. Bob Herbert, "Mugged in the Hospital," *New York Times*, August 9, 1996, A27.

8. *Consumer Reports*, 61 (1996), 28, 31, 38. These stories appear with astonishing frequency. See, for yet more examples, Stuart Auerbach, "Managed Care Backlash," *Washington Post*, June 25, 1996, Z12.

9. Council on Ethical and Judicial Affairs, American Medical Association, "Ethical Issues in Managed Care," *JAMA*, 273 (1995), 330–35.

10. Kathleen T. Smith, "Managed Care Safeguards Sought by States," *Nursing Economics*, 13 (1995), 312; Christine Van Dusen, "State Ranks Among Best for HMO Grievances," *Business Today*, July 27, 1996, 1C.

11. Richard A. Knox, "State Legislatures Take On HMOs' Managed Care Policies," *Boston Globe*, July 24, 1996, A12. The HMO response has often been to claim that the flurry of legislation is inspired not by patients to protect their interests but by physicians to protect their incomes.

12. Milt Freudenheim, "H.M.O.'s Cope with a Backlash on Cost Cutting," *New York Times*, May 19, 1996, 1.

13. Allison Bell, "HMOs and PPOs Rate Their Legislative Priorities," *National Underwriter*, July 15, 1996, 6.

14. *Wall Street Journal*, August 2, 1996, 28. To be sure, the costs to individuals may not be reduced to the extent that they want interventions not covered by HMOs. Accordingly, some physicians are busily recruiting patients for cosmetic surgery and infertility treatments; because these services are not covered by the HMOs, doctors can charge what the traffic will bear.

15. John E. Billi et al., "Potential Effects of Managed Care on Specialty Practice at a University Medical Center," *NEJM*, 333 (1995), 979–83.

16. Dolores G. Clement et al., "Access and Outcomes of Elderly Patients Enrolled in Managed Care," *JAMA*, 271 (1994), 1490.

17. Miller and Luft, "Managed Care Plan Performance," 1515, 1517; N. R. Every et al., "Resource Utilization in the Treatment of Acute Myocardial Infarction," *Journal of the American College of Cardiology*, 26 (1995), 401–6, and editorial comment by Harlan M. Krumholz, 407–8. There are also some suggestive findings that HMO physicians differ from their colleagues when responding to hypothetical cases, more prepared to use less expensive interventions. Thus it may be that the HMO affects the mind-set of its physicians, making them more conscious than they might even realize to the role of costs in selecting health care interventions. Daniel S. Lessler and Andrew L. Avins, "Cost, Uncertainty, and Doctors' Decisions: The Case of Thrombolytic Therapy," *Archives of Internal Medicine*, 152 (1992), 1665–72.

18. Miller and Luft, "Managed Care Plan Performance," 1514.

19. John Rapoport, Stephen Gehlbach, Stanley Lemeshow, and Daniel Teres, "Resource Utilization among Intensive Care Patients," *Archives of Internal Medicine*, 152 (1992), 2211.

20. Miller and Luft, "Managed Care Plan Performance," 1516.

21. Karen Davis et al., "Choice Matters: Enrollees' View of Their Health Plans," *Health Affairs*, 14 (1995), 105.

22. Safran et al., "Primary Care Performance," 1585.

23. Davis et al., "Choice Matters," 105.

24. Wall Street research reports on HMOs are hedging their bets, noting that HMO operating margins are now very low but that patient recruitment is increasing and managerial skills are improving.

25. Safran et al., "Primary Care Performance," 1579. But for an opposing view, see Ellen Coffey et al., "Capitated Medicaid and the Process of Care of Elderly Hypertensives and Diabetics," *American Journal of Medicine*, 98 (1995), 531.

Index